SOFT FOOD IDEAS *for* DINNER

Recipes and food ideas
for after Dental Procedures,
Wisdom Tooth Removal,
Tooth extractions or
dental sensitivity.

By Suzanne Burke

SOFT FOOD IDEAS *for* DINNER

© **2024 Copyright Suzanne Burke. All rights reserved.**
No part of this publication may be, stored in a retrieval system or transmitted in any form by any means, electronic or mechanical, recording, scanning or otherwise without the prior written permission of the author

Paperback ISBN 978-0-6483205-4-8

SOFT FOOD IDEAS *for* DINNER

Disclaimer – Important PLEASE READ

The information presented within this book is the author's opinion and does not constitute any health or medical advice. The content of this book is for informational purposes only.

Please seek advice from your healthcare provider for your personal health concerns prior to acting on any of the information in this book.
This book is not a replacement for advice from your orthodontist, dentist, dietician or any other health professional. All recipes and food recommendations have been made with the purpose of providing you with fun and interesting food ideas and for general information purposes only.

Dietary recommendations are healthy for the majority of people but potentially dangerous for others. You are responsible for your own health and safety at all times. By continuing to read this book beyond this page you acknowledge and agree to the above and the following:

- You have been assessed and are under the care of a qualified professional for your braces and dental health management.
- You are responsible for your own diet choices. In particular, if you have any special dietary needs or medical conditions that require a special diet, that you have consulted a health professional.
- This book does not provide medical advice. Where there is a conflict between the information in this book and the advice provided by your health care provider(s), then the advice of the health care provider should be followed.
- All material provided in this book and associated website, including text, images, graphics, photos and anything else, are all provides for informational purposes only are not a substitute for medical advice or treatment.
- You acknowledge and understand that sugar can be harmful to your teeth and consuming too much sugar can lead to build of plaque on your teeth & lead to teeth decay. You are responsible for ensuring that you consume sugar in moderation. If in doubt as to what is an acceptable level of sugar in your diet, consult a health professional to seek advice.
- The author and or publishers are not responsible for any recipes that you cook that fail! While every effort has gone into providing high quality content, even the simplest of recipes can fail!

Table of Contents

INTRODUCTION v
WHY THIS BOOK WAS WRITTEN 1
WHO IS THIS BOOK FOR? 1
WHAT YOU WILL GET OUT OF THIS BOOK 1
DISCLAIMER: WHAT THIS BOOK IS NOT 2
THE FIRST WEEK AFTER A DENTAL PROCEDURE 3
WHAT TO EAT AFTER THE FIRST WEEK 8
BREAKFAST FOOD IDEAS 8
LUNCH IDEAS 9
DINNER IDEAS 10
DESSERT IDEAS 10
SNACKS FOR EATING ON THE RUN OR QUICK BITES 11
MAKING GREAT SOFT FOOD CHOICES 15
TEMPTING FUSSY EATERS 19
BREAKFAST IDEAS AND RECIPES 20
LUNCH AND DINNER RECIPES 31
DESSERT RECIPES 59
EASY LUNCHBOX SOLUTIONS 72
MODIFYING COMMON RECIPES FOR SOFT FOOD MEALS 75
TIPS FOR EATING OUT AND ORDERING TAKE-AWAY ... 78
SAMPLE MEAL PLAN - FIRST WEEK 89
SAMPLE MEAL PLAN – AFTER FIRST WEEK 90
ABOUT THE AUTHOR 91

SOFT FOOD IDEAS *for* DINNER

Introduction

This is a helpful guide designed to make your meals both delicious and easy to manage when you need to be eating soft food. Whether you've just had dental surgery, tooth extraction, or any major oral procedure, this book is here to help you navigate your dietary needs. When your teeth and gums are feeling sensitive, you will need some food options that are easy to eat. This book provides options for a range of soft food options. Some will not require any chewing at all such as soups and smoothies and these are perfect for when you are feeling the most sensitive.

There is also a wide range of options and ideas for when your teeth have settled, but you still require relatively soft food to prevent pain or discomfort.

My aim is to provide you with a variety of recipes and food ideas that are soft, nutritious, and easy to prepare.

Food For Sensitive Gums

Nearly all the food in this book is non-spicy and non-acidic. This means that sore gums and ulcers in your mouth will not sting or feel uncomfortable when eating.

Non-Staining Food

Dentures, crowns and braces (particularly ceramic) can stain easily with certain types of food. I have included many recommendations for food to avoid and better still, lots of options for food that won't cause staining issues.

Getting Food Stuck

You will need to avoid food that will get stuck in your extraction site, or in your braces as this may lead to infection, tooth decay and other problems. This book includes tips for food to avoid such as small seeds and nuts.

SOFT FOOD IDEAS *for* DINNER

Why This Book Was Written

The idea for this book was born out of the need to provide practical, enjoyable meal solutions for those recovering from oral surgery. After undergoing dental procedures, it can be challenging to find foods that are gentle on your mouth yet satisfying. This book addresses that gap, offering a range of recipes that are not only easy to eat but also delicious and varied.

Who Is This Book For?

This book is suitable for anyone on a soft food diet. This may be after having wisdom teeth removed or after a dental procedure, a tooth extractions or perhaps you just have sensitive teeth. The reasons for needing a soft food diet are many and could include:

- Dental/oral surgery or procedure
- Wisdom tooth removal
- Tooth extractions
- Dental braces – what to eat the first week and after adjustments
- Dental sensitivity
- Anyone needing a soft food diet, whatever your reason may be!

What You Will Get Out of This Book

In this book, you'll find:

- Easy-to-follow recipes for soft, tasty meals
- Meal planning ideas
- Creative food options to prevent mealtime boredom
- What foods you should avoid

SOFT FOOD IDEAS *for* DINNER

Disclaimer: What this book is not

This book is not a replacement for advice from your orthodontist, dentist, dietician or any other health professional. All recipes and food recommendations have been made with the purpose of providing you with fun and interesting food ideas. This means that the food and recipes are not necessarily nutritionally balanced! Please seek professional advice if you have special needs such as food allergies, diabetes, gluten intolerance or any medical condition where your diet is important.

Please remember:

- √ This book has NOT been written by a medical or health professional.
- √ This book and contents are NOT medical or health advice and do not replace professional health advice.
- √ Recipes in this book are meant to be yummy and are NOT necessarily nutritionally balanced.
- √ Seek professional advice if you have special dietary requirements.
- √ If there is a conflict between medical advice and contents in this book, then the MEDICAL ADVICE SHOULD BE FOLLOWED.

SOFT FOOD IDEAS for DINNER

The First Week After a Dental Procedure

In the first week after a dental procedure, it is a good idea to focus on foods that require minimal or no chewing to avoid irritation and ensure proper healing.

What to Eat in the First Week

The first week post-procedure can be a period of adjustment for most people. There will likely be some discomfort as your mouth heals. During the first few days, or even the entire first week, you may want to avoid chewing altogether.
Pureed foods, which can be spooned in without chewing, will be your best options. Although this might sound unappetizing at first, there are plenty of delicious and nutritious options like smoothies, soups, and more.

Introducing More Variety

As the days go by, you can gradually introduce soft foods with a bit more substance, and eventually, more solid foods that require minimal chewing. Before long, you'll be able to eat normally again.
However, it is important to be cautious and avoid foods that could cause discomfort or disrupt the healing process. Remember, this is just a temporary phase, and focusing on what you can eat rather than what you can't, will make this period more enjoyable. Get creative in the kitchen and try some of the ideas listed here.

SOFT FOOD IDEAS *for* DINNER

Food Ideas for the First Week

Store-Bought Options:

- Ice-cream
- Chocolate mousse
- Crème caramel
- Jelly
- Custard
- Pre-made smooth soups (or puree them yourself)

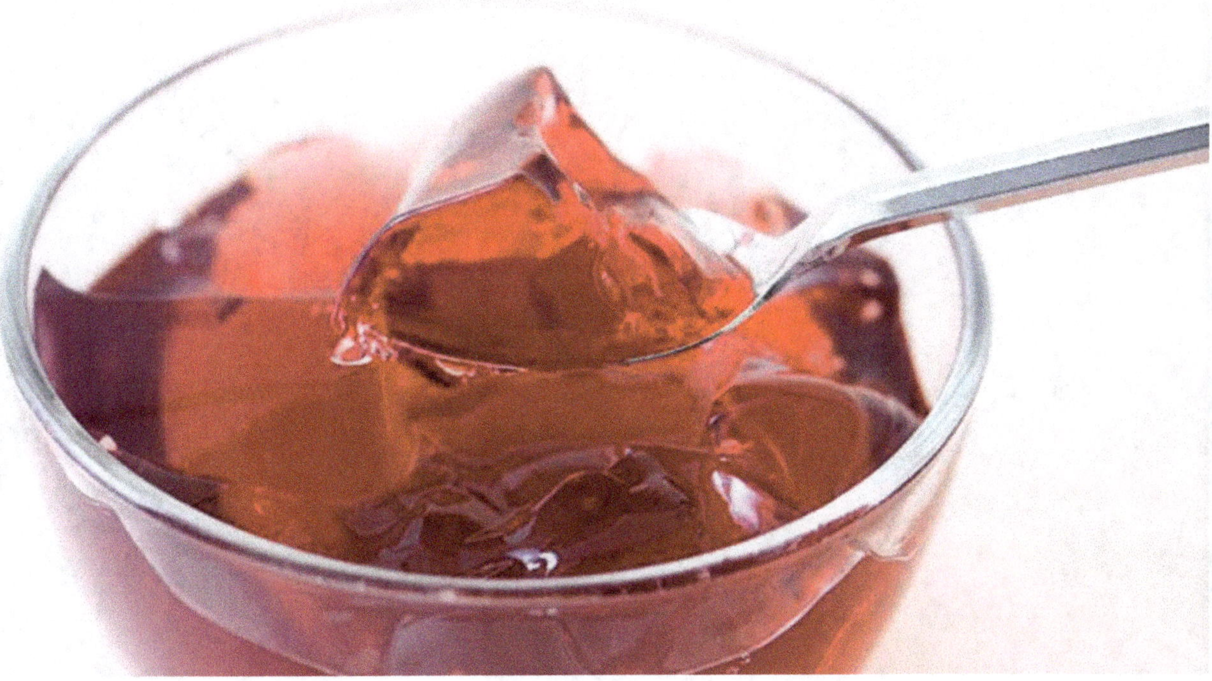

SOFT FOOD IDEAS *for* DINNER

Breakfast Ideas

- Soft, stewed, or mashed fruit (e.g., apples, bananas)
- Smoothies (strawberry, blueberry, vanilla, mango, banana)
- Scrambled eggs
- Yogurt
- Porridge
- Softened cereal

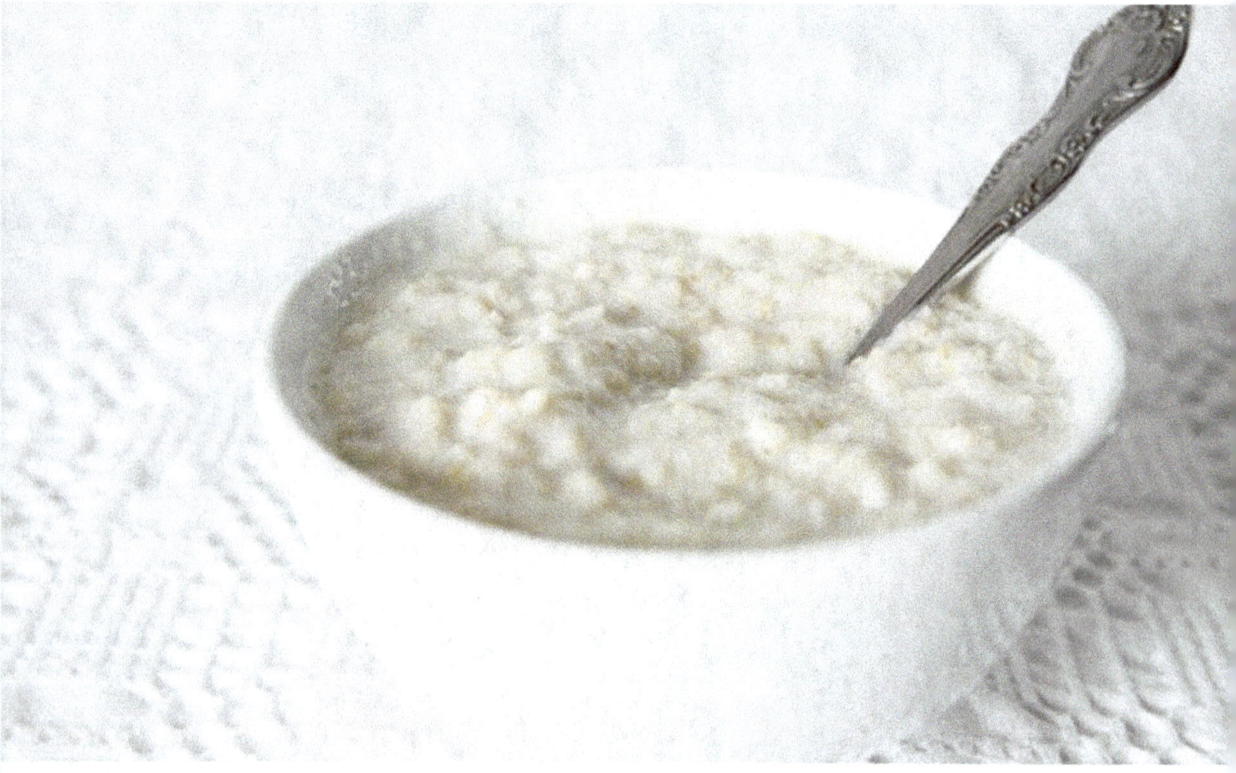

SOFT FOOD IDEAS *for* DINNER

Lunch and Dinner Ideas

- Soups (potato, vegetable, pumpkin, chicken noodle)
- Fish chowder
- Mashed potatoes with gravy and mushrooms
- Fish patties
- Salmon and pea pasta
- Roasted vegetables (soft only, not fibrous)
- Mild Mexican beans
- Chicken and corn chowder
- Meatloaf
- Pulled pork
- Baked or poached fish
- Steamed or boiled vegetables (with added butter, salt, and pepper to taste)

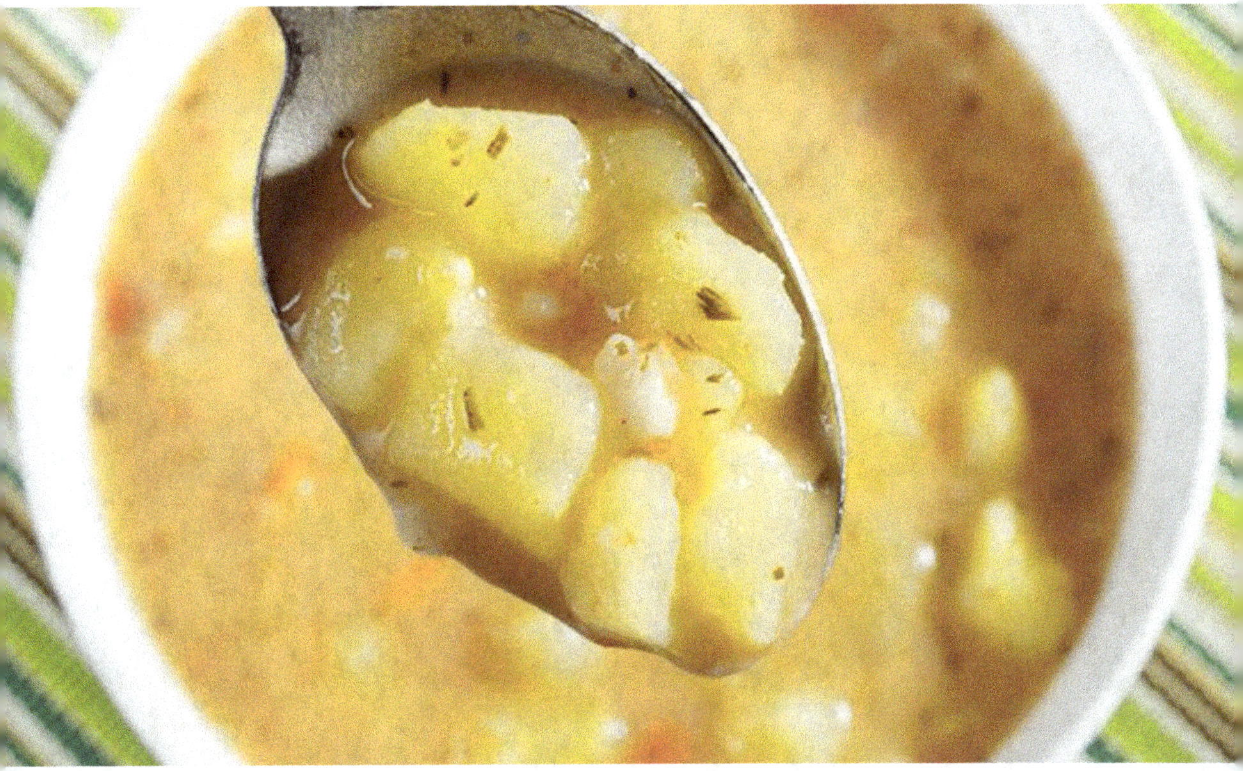

SOFT FOOD IDEAS *for* DINNER

Dessert Ideas

- Ice cream (no nuts)
- Jelly
- Custard
- Chocolate mousse
- Pannacotta

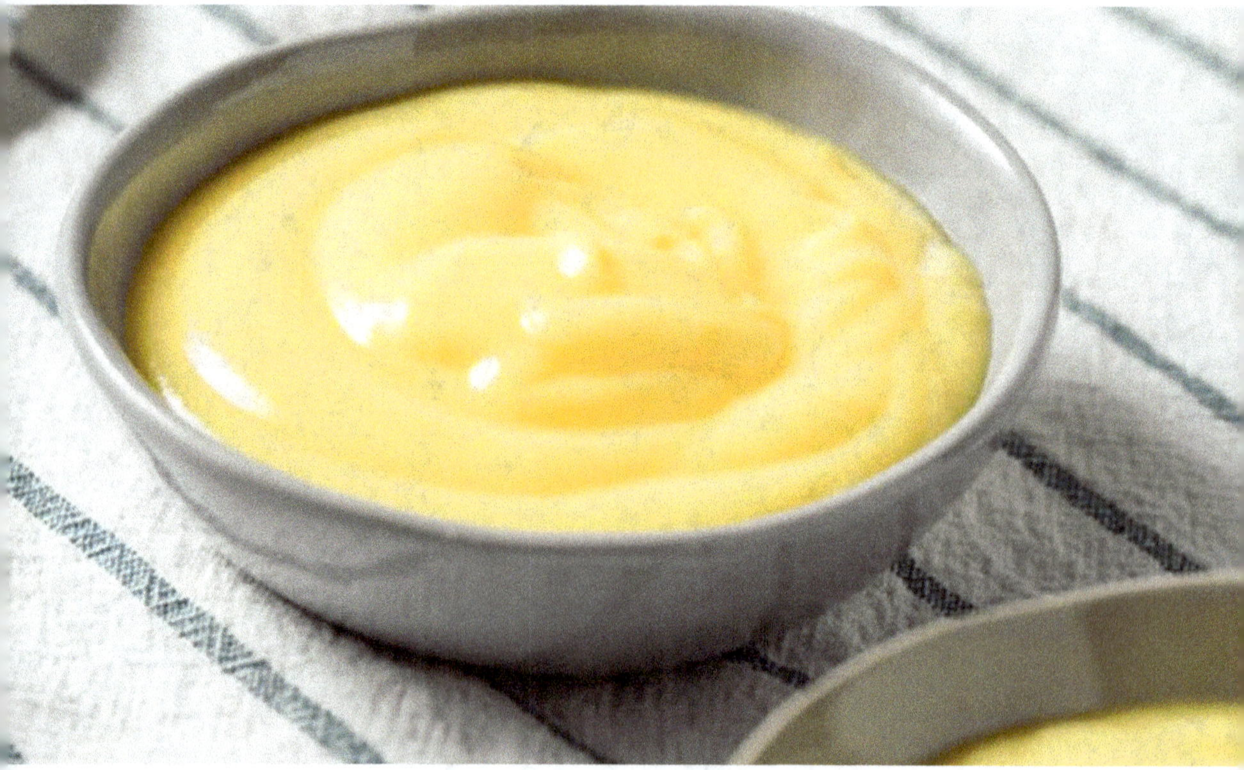

SOFT FOOD IDEAS *for* DINNER

What to Eat After the First Week

As your mouth continues to heal, you can start incorporating a wider variety of soft foods into your diet. Here are some ideas that should be easy to eat and gentle on your recovering mouth.

Breakfast Food Ideas

- **Pancakes:** Light and fluffy, pancakes are a perfect post-surgery breakfast.
- **French Toast:** Made with soft bread, thoroughly soaked in an egg mixture and cooked until tender.
- **Toast without Crusts:** Top with soft toppings like mushrooms and sour cream.
- **Mashed Avocado on Soft Bread:** Use soft bread like brioche for a creamy and delicious meal.
- **Muffins:** Soft and moist, perfect for breakfast or a snack.
- **Waffles:** Light and easy to chew, served with soft toppings like fruit puree.

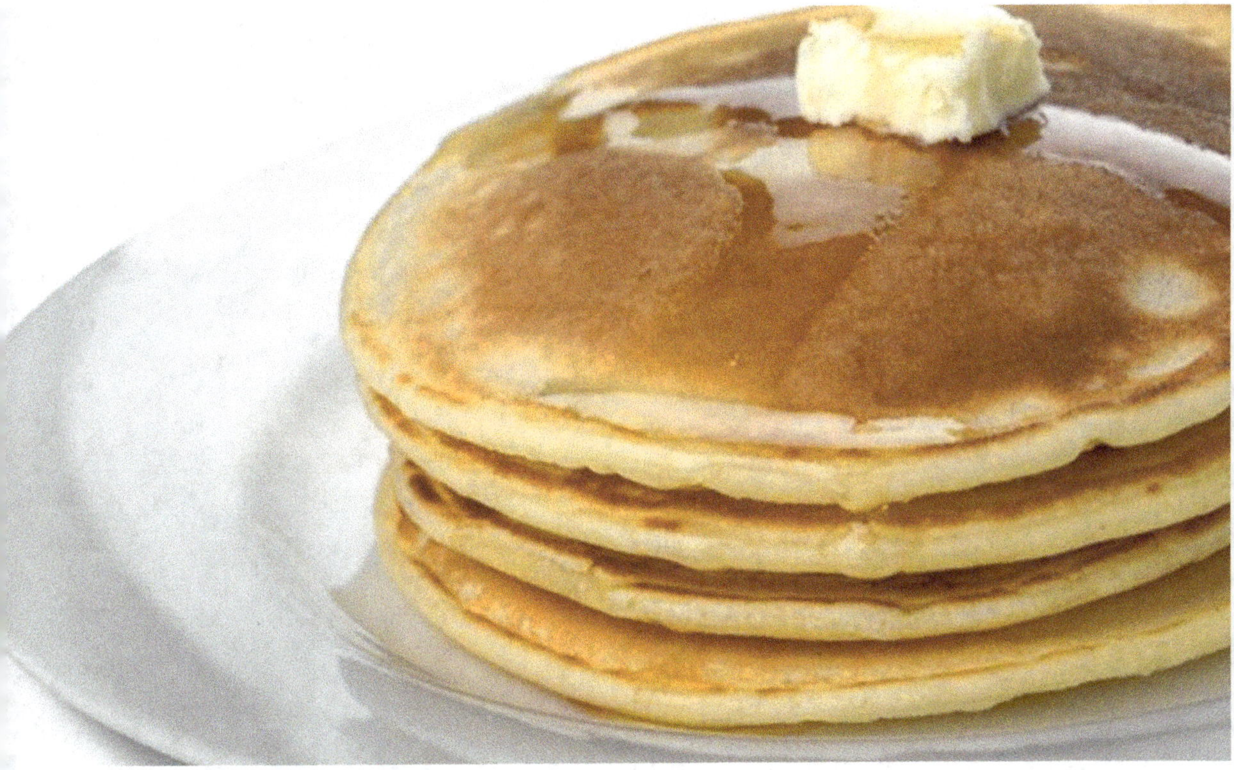

SOFT FOOD IDEAS *for* DINNER

Lunch Ideas

1. Soft Bread Sandwiches (No Crusts): Fill with chopped boiled egg, thinly sliced ham and tomato, or hummus.
2. Potato Salad: Soft and creamy, an excellent lunch option.
3. Macaroni Cheese: Soft pasta in a creamy cheese sauce.

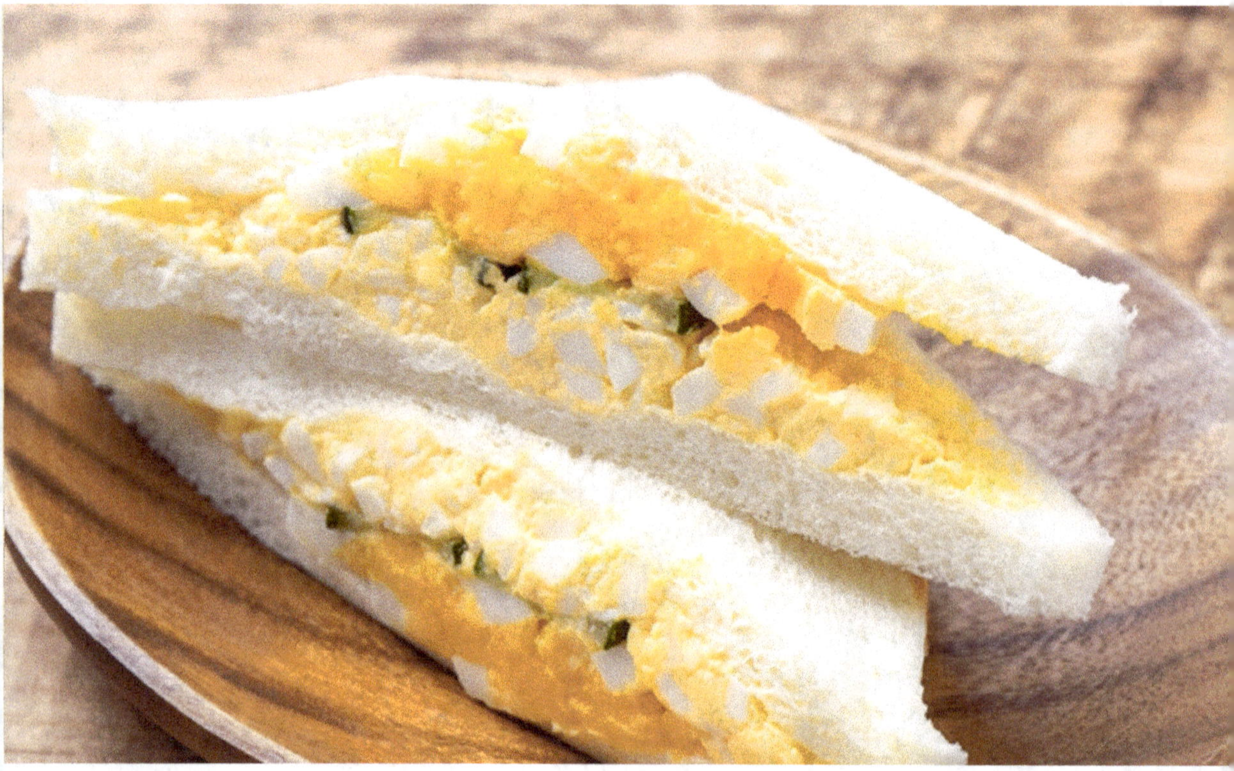

SOFT FOOD IDEAS *for* DINNER

Dinner Ideas

1. **Protein Sources:** Soft options like lentils, beans, tofu, fish, chicken, and slow-cooked meat.
2. **Pasta Bake:** Soft pasta in a rich, creamy sauce.
3. **Shepherd's Pie / Cottage Pie:** Soft mashed potatoes with a hearty filling.
4. **Chicken Pie:** Soft pastry filled with tender chicken and vegetables.
5. **Pan-Fried Salmon with Sweet Potato Mash:** A nutritious and soft dinner option.
6. **Filled Pasta:** Ravioli or tortellini with a creamy sauce.
7. **Soft Noodles:** Egg noodles, udon, or rice noodles.
8. **Soft Nachos:** Use cut-up pita bread instead of corn chips.
9. **Slow-Cooked Meat:** Tender options like lamb shanks or pulled pork.
10. **Risotto:** Creamy and soft rice dish.

Salad and Vegetables

1. **Shredded Lettuce:** Soft and easy to chew.
2. **Guacamole:** Creamy avocado dip.
3. **Boiled and Steamed Vegetables:** Cooked until very soft.
4. **Mashed Potatoes:** A staple soft food.
5. **Potato Salad:** Soft and creamy.
6. **Pasta Salad:** Use soft pasta and mild ingredients.
7. **Cauliflower Cheese:** Soft cauliflower in a cheesy sauce.

Dessert Ideas

1. **Apple Crumble:** Soft baked apples with a crumbly topping.
2. **Custard and Strawberries:** Smooth custard with soft, sweet strawberries.
3. **Jelly, Custard, Chocolate Mousse Layer Sundae:** A layered dessert of soft treats.
4. **Trifle in a Cup:** Sponge cake with custard.
5. **Chocolate Cake:** Moist and soft.
6. **Chocolate Pudding:** Rich and creamy.
7. **Chocolate Mousse:** Light and airy.

SOFT FOOD IDEAS *for* DINNER

Snacks for Eating on the Run or Quick Bites

1. **Muffins:** Flavors like pear and dark chocolate.
2. **Soft Fruit:** Options like kiwi, banana, rockmelon, and seedless grapes.
3. **Chocolate Pudding:** Easy to eat and delicious.
4. **Cake and Cupcakes:** Soft and moist varieties.
5. **Carrot and Apple Cake:** Made without nuts.
6. **Ice-Cream:** Smooth and soothing.
7. **Soft Cookies:** Gentle on the teeth.
8. **Hash Browns:** Soft and crispy.
9. **Apple Sauce:** Smooth and sweet.
10. **Bananas:** Easy to eat and nutritious.

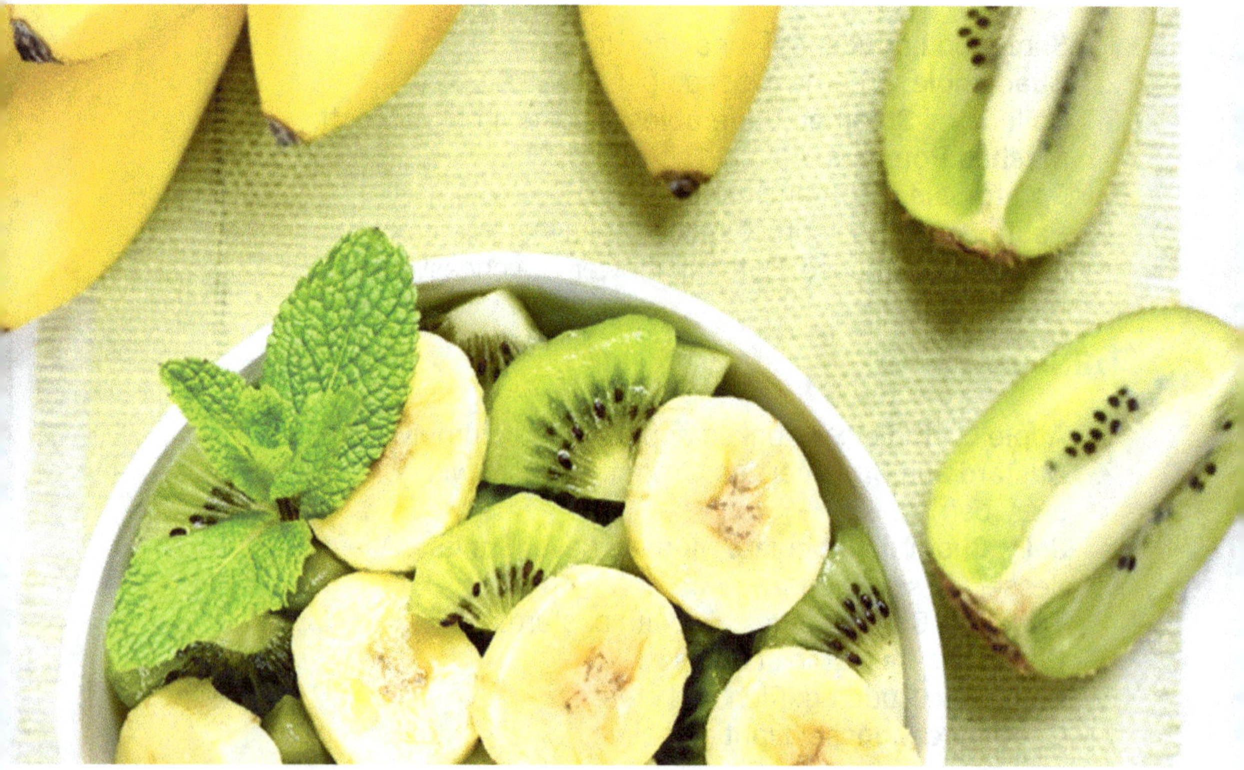

SOFT FOOD IDEAS *for* DINNER

Types of Foods to Avoid

After a dental procedure, certain foods can hinder the healing process or cause discomfort. It's essential to avoid these types of foods to ensure a smooth recovery.

Avoiding Hard or Crunchy Foods

Hard or crunchy foods can damage healing tissues and cause pain. Avoid these:
- Corn chips
- Nuts, Granola, Muesli
- Popcorn
- Raw vegetables (like carrots)

Avoiding Sticky or Chewy Foods

Sticky foods can be difficult to remove and may cause discomfort. Avoid these:
- Chewing gum
- Toffees
- Caramels
- Sticky candies

Avoiding Small Seeds and Grains

Tiny seeds and grains can get stuck and irritate healing tissues. Avoid these:
- Poppy seeds
- Sesame seeds
- Quinoa

Avoiding Spicy Foods

Spicy foods can exacerbate irritation and pain in the mouth. Avoid these:
- Curries
- Foods containing chili
- Acidic foods like lemon juice dressings

SOFT FOOD IDEAS for DINNER

Big Bite Foods

Foods that require large bites can strain your mouth and cause healing issues. Avoid these or cut into small, manageable pieces:
- Hamburgers
- Hotdogs
- Apples
- Corn on the cob
- Ribs

Staining Foods

Foods that can stain teeth and dental work should be avoided to maintain oral hygiene. Examples include:
- Berries: Blueberries, raspberries, blackberries
- Yellow curries
- Beetroot
- Black coffee, tea (weak or herbal tea is okay)
- Red wine
- Rich tomato-based sauces
- Strongly pigmented spices: Turmeric, paprika

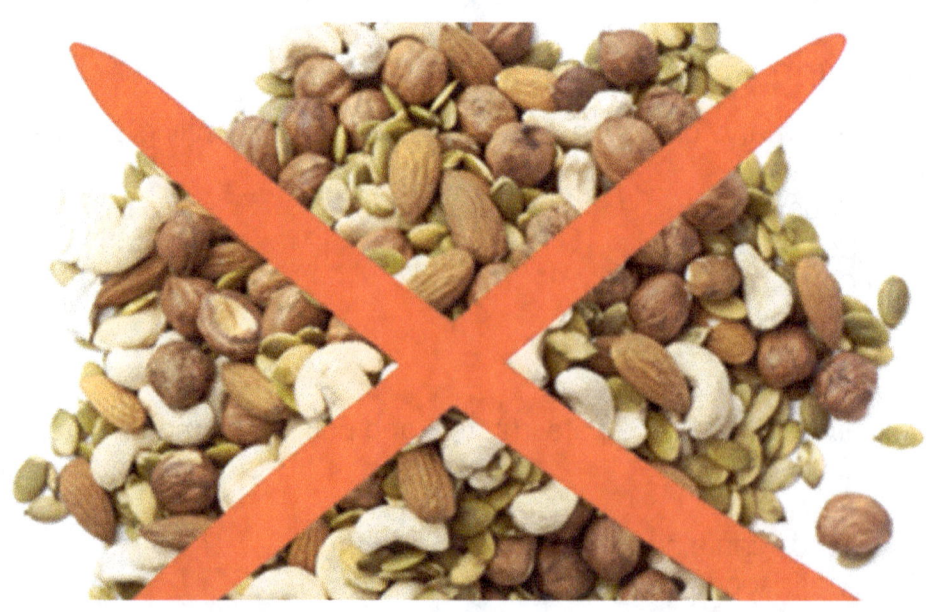

SOFT FOOD IDEAS *for* DINNER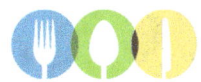

Non-Food Things to avoid chewing on

- Avoid chewing the end of your pen or pen lid
- Do Not bite your fingernails!
- Do not crunch on ice!

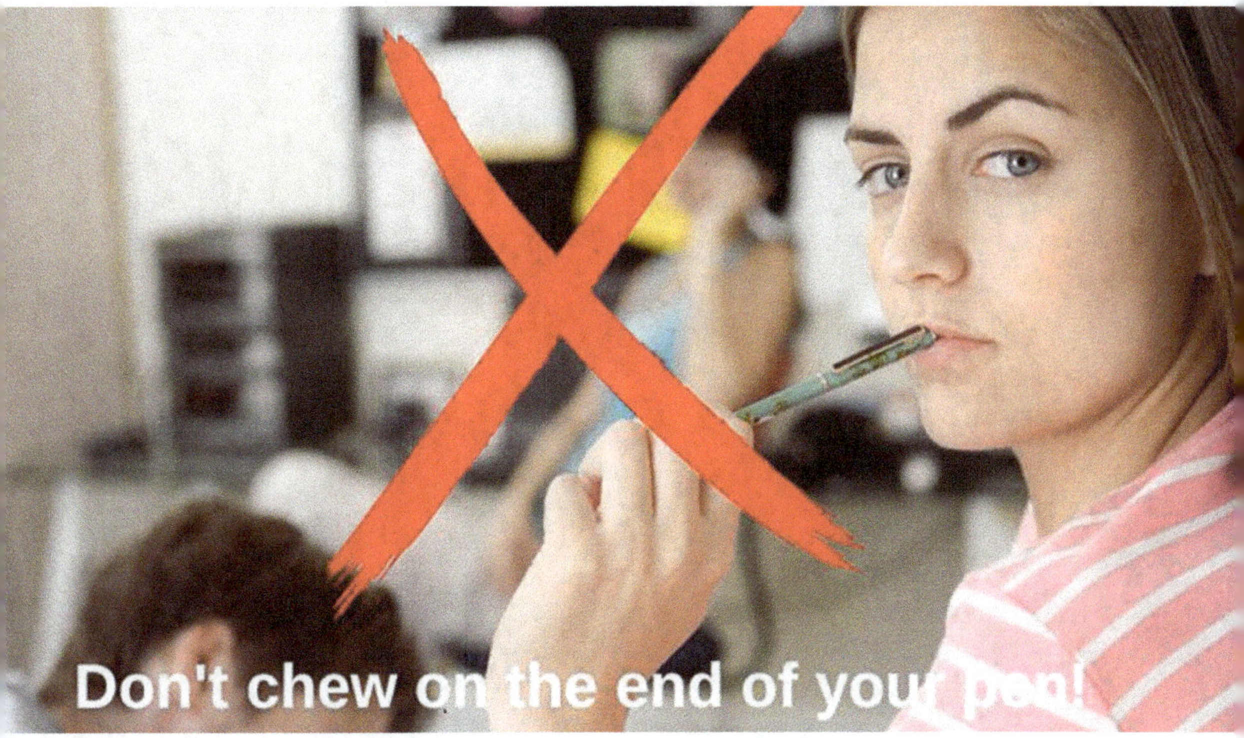

Don't chew on the end of your pen!

SOFT FOOD IDEAS for DINNER

Making Great Soft Food Choices

Even when eating soft food, you will be able to eat relatively 'normal' food. Make life easy for yourself and aim to eat food that will not require too much chewing to minimise the stress on your mouth and teeth.

Meat and Protein

Great sources of easy to eat protein include chicken, tofu, beans, fish and eggs. Red meat is fine but should be tender and/or cut into small pieces.

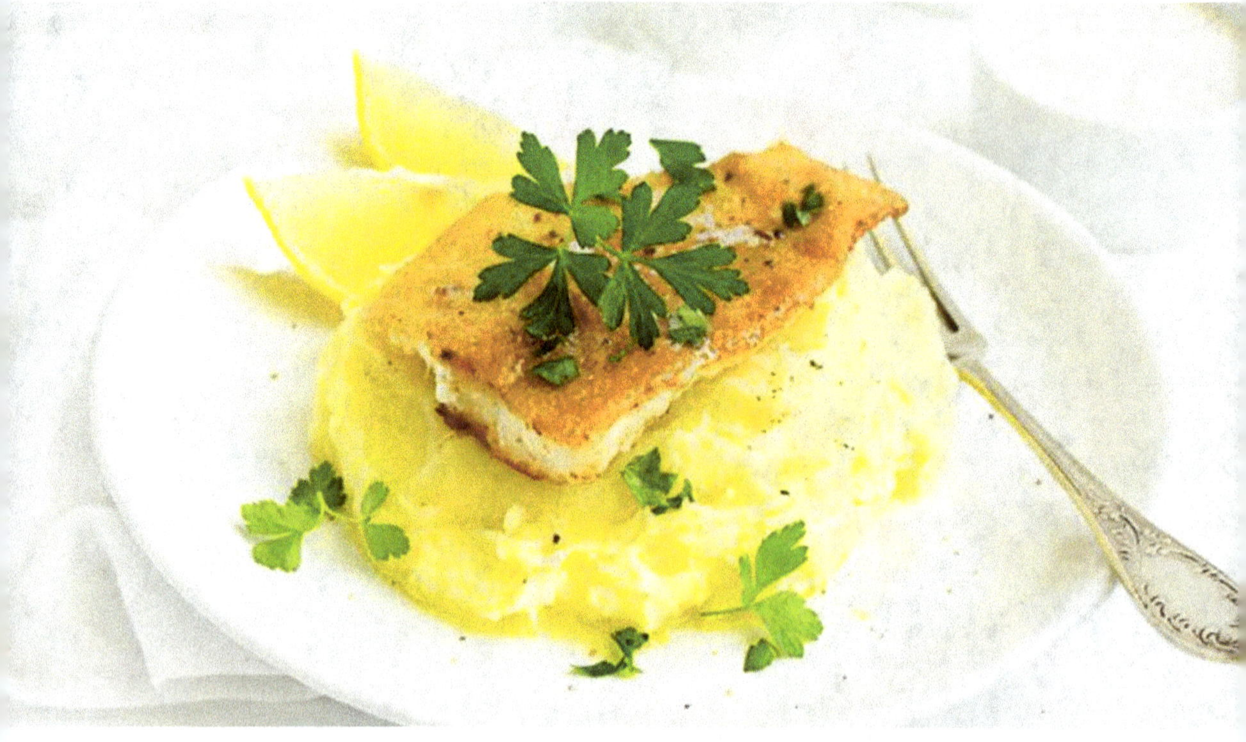

SOFT FOOD IDEAS *for* DINNER

Vegetables

Vegetables can be your friend and mashed potatoes is an all- time favourite, though most vegetables are ok as long as they are cooked until soft.

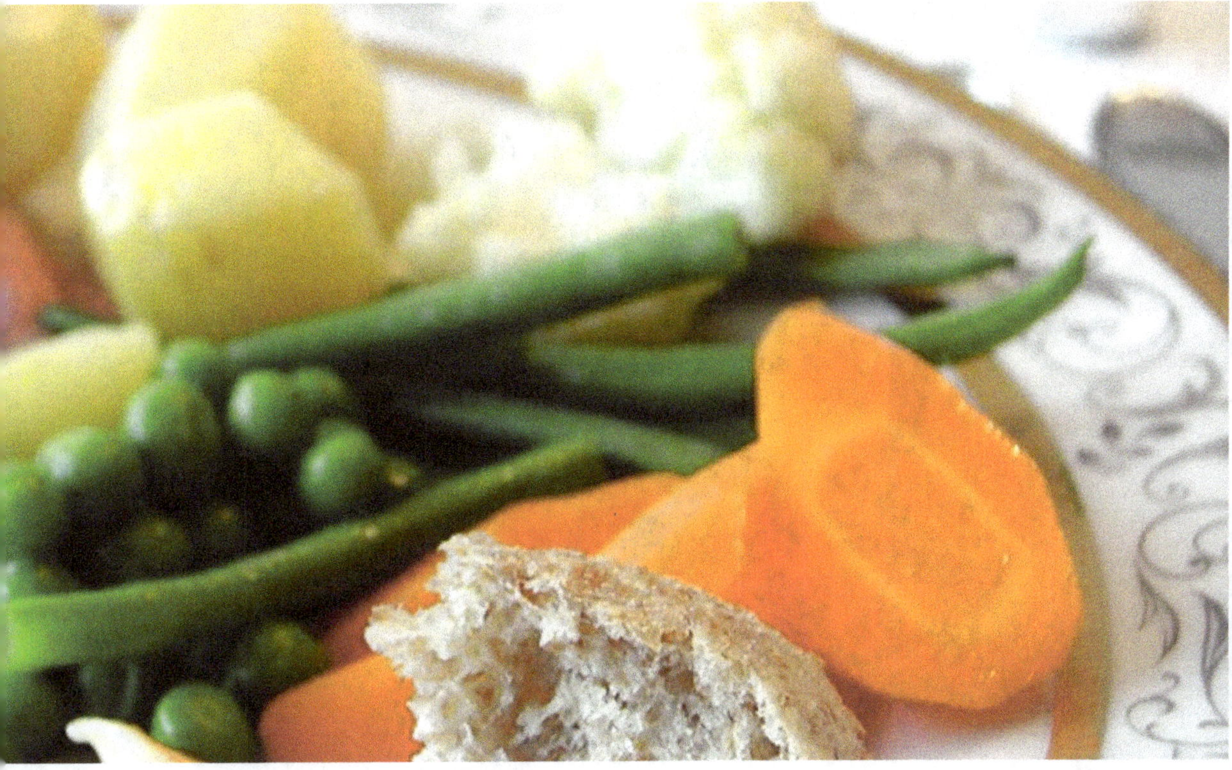

SOFT FOOD IDEAS *for* DINNER

Fruit

Eating fruit is still ok, you just need to adapt a bit by cutting fruit into small bite size pieces or choose soft fruit such as bananas.

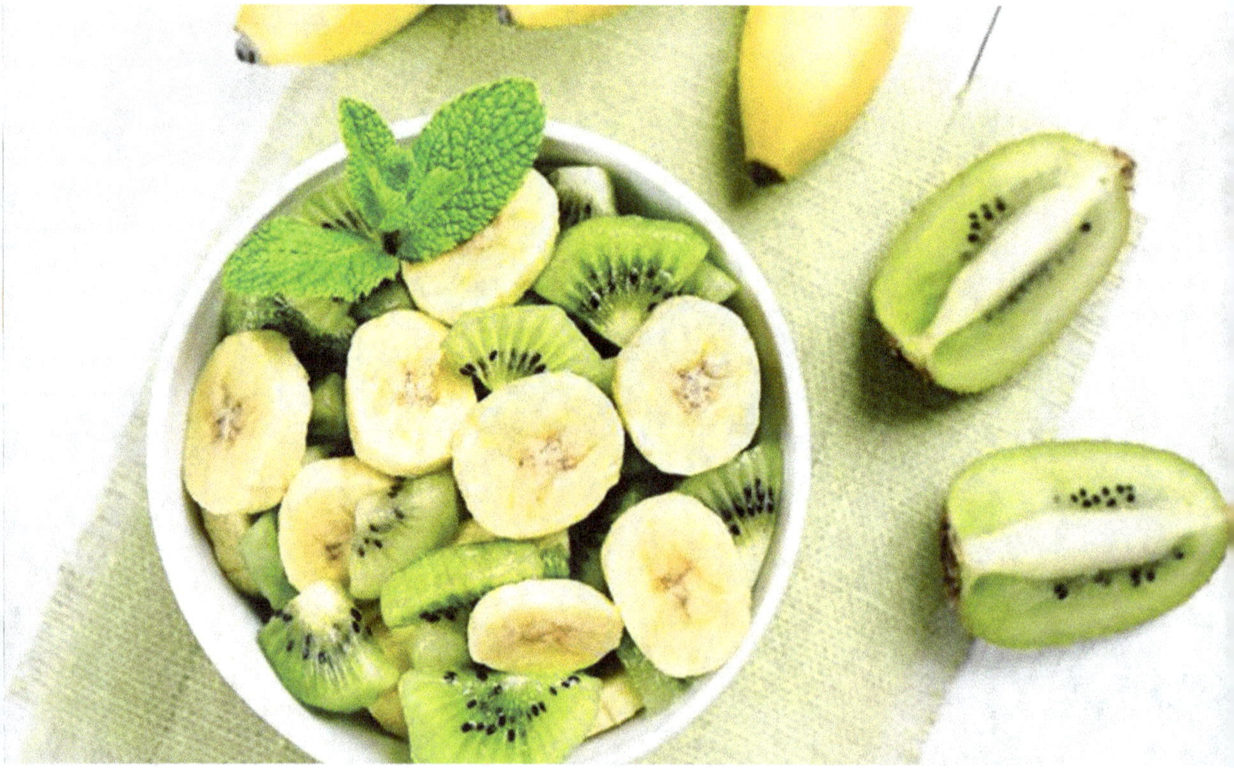

SOFT FOOD IDEAS *for* DINNER

Carbohydrates

Pasta and soft bread are the best options. You can eat rice and other grains too, but you will find that the saml pieces may be something to watch for.

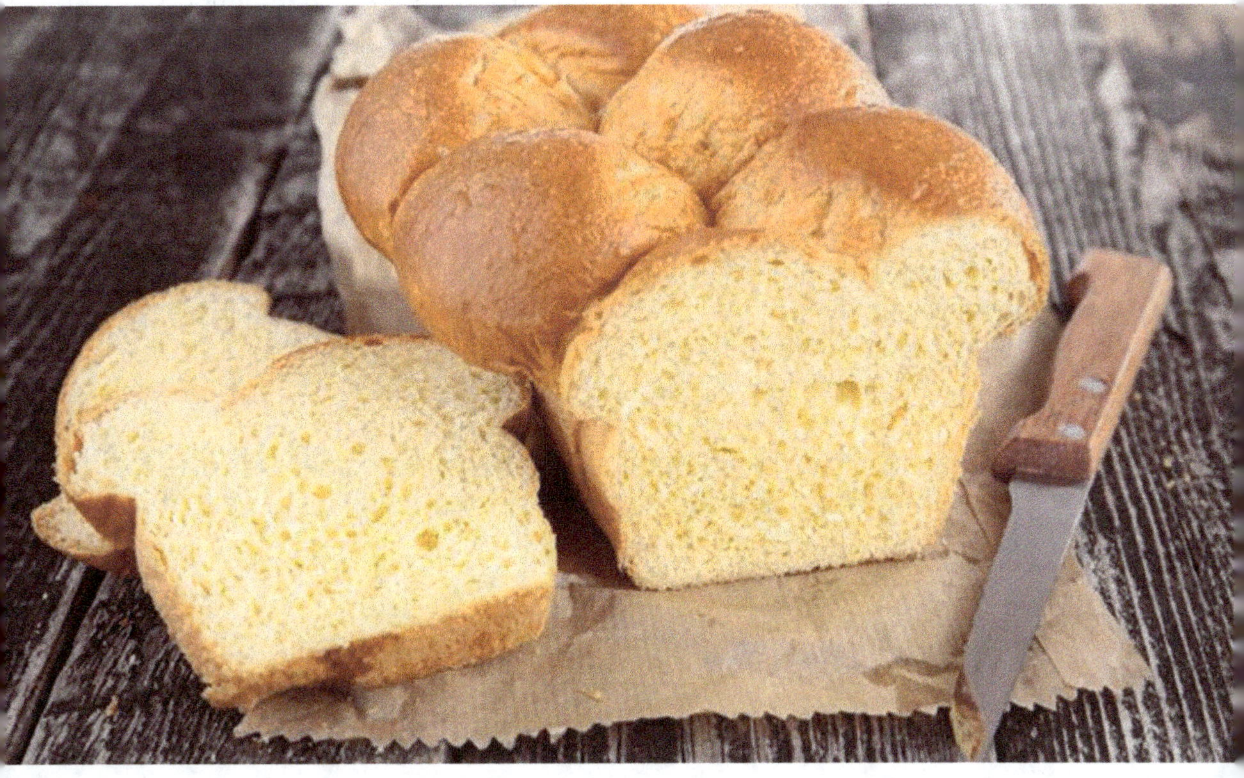

SOFT FOOD IDEAS for DINNER

Tempting Fussy Eaters

Mealtimes should be harmonious, not a battleground. Whether you are cooking for yourself, or for elderly loved one, or someone recovering from dental surgery, it can be challenging to make meals appealing. Here are some strategies to tempt even the fussiest of eaters, ensuring that mealtime remains a pleasant and stress-free experience.

Winning Ideas to Help Tempt Fussy Eaters

Give Ownership: Allow individuals to have a say in what they eat. Let them help decide what to buy, what to cook, and what to have for dinner.

Involve Them in Shopping: Take them to the store – if it is possible to do so - and let them choose a couple of items they would like to try. This involvement can make them more interested in eating the food they selected.

Respect Preferences: Acknowledge and respect that everyone has food preferences. Encourage trying new foods, but don't force anyone to eat something they truly dislike.

Educational Approach: Share information about the nutritional benefits of different foods and how they contribute to overall health. Avoid Pressure: Never force or pressure someone to eat a particular food. Encourage and offer but let them decide.

Be Patient: It can take several attempts before someone starts to enjoy a new food. Encourage them to try a few bites on different occasions without making it a big deal.

SOFT FOOD IDEAS *for* DINNER

Breakfast Ideas and Recipes

Apple Puree - perfect soft food

Ingredients
- 2 Pink Lady or Granny Smith apples
- ½ tsp raw sugar (optional)
- Splash of water

Method
1. Peel and core the apple, then finely chop.
2. Place chopped apple, sugar and a splash of water into a small pot on medium heat.
3. Cook for 5 minutes or until tender.
4. Use a fork to mash or a stick blender to puree.
5. Serve warm or cold.

Tip: make a big batch & freeze in portions and defrost one or two after each adjustment.

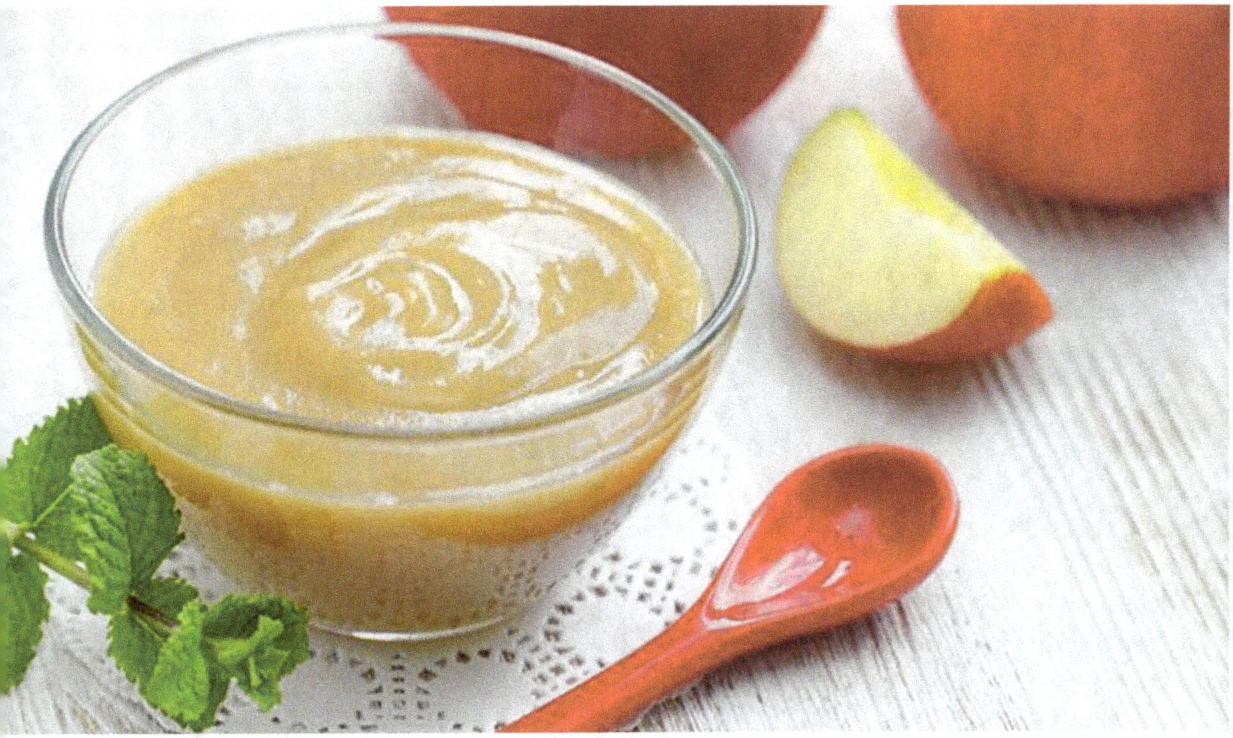

SOFT FOOD IDEAS *for* DINNER

Banana and Cinnamon mash - fast and easy

Ingredients
- 1 Banana
- Sprinkle of cinnamon

Method
1. Peel and roughly chop banana into a bowl and mash with a fork.
2. Dust with cinnamon and enjoy.

Tip: this can also be used as the base for a simple smoothie, just add a cup of milk and whizz up in a blender.

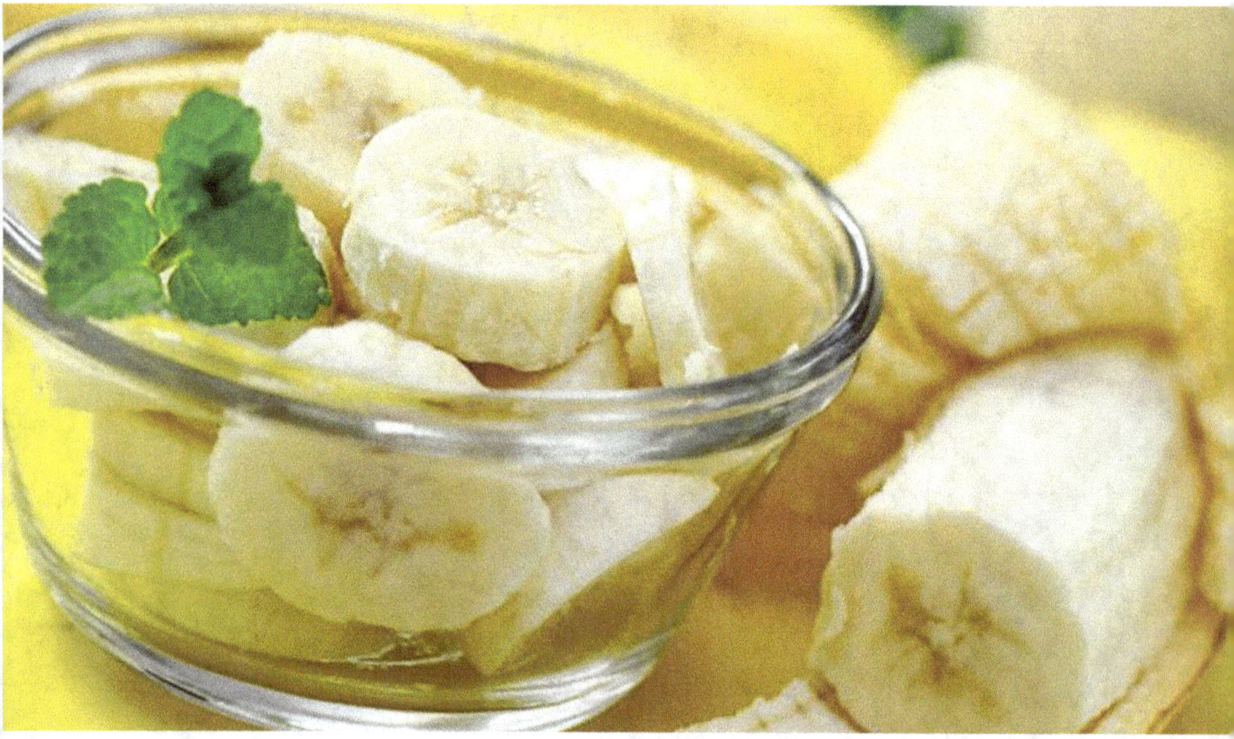

SOFT FOOD IDEAS *for* DINNER

Breakfast Smoothies!!!

About smoothies: these are a wonderful way to get a filling and nutritious meal or snack without the need to chew at all. Absolutely perfect for anytime when your teeth or gums are sore or just need a break.

Basic Ingredients
- ¾ cup of your chosen milk – cow, almond, oat, rice
- 1 scoop of vanilla protein powder (optional)
- Add your choice of fruit

Method
1. Add all ingredients to a blender and whizz!

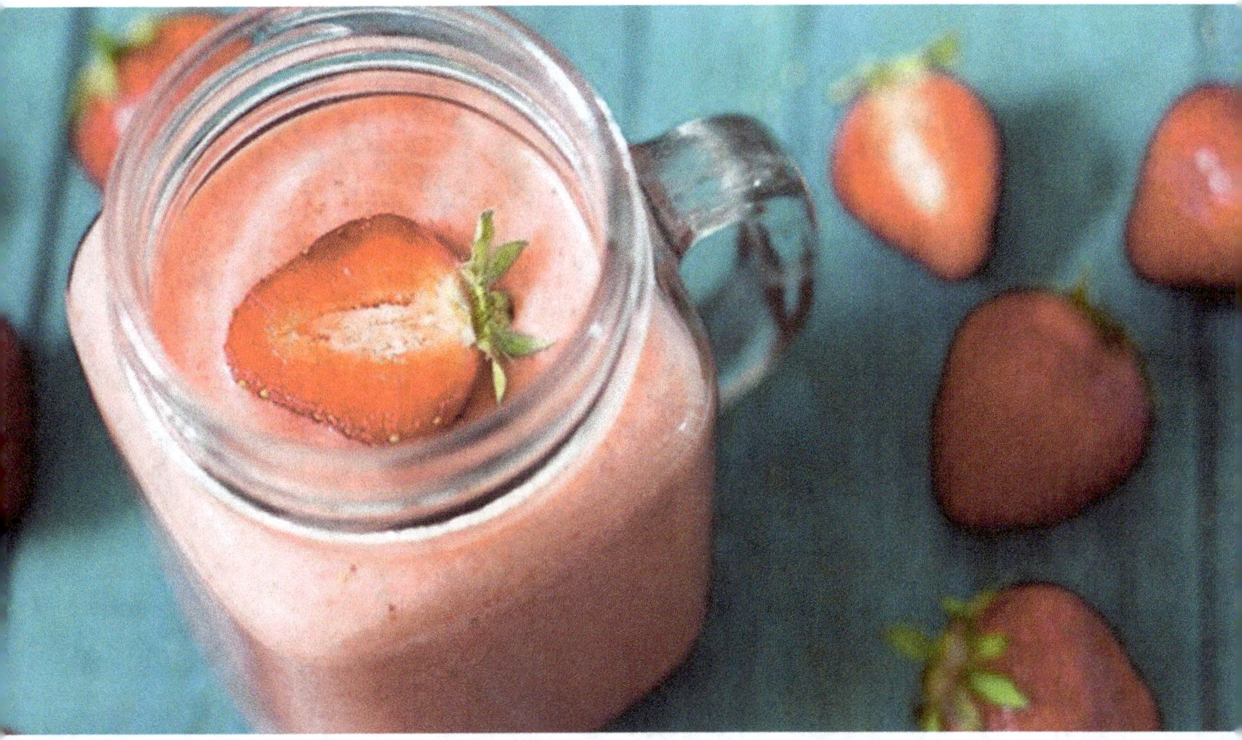

SOFT FOOD IDEAS *for* DINNER

Breakfast Smoothies!!!
All the Colours of the RAINBOW!

- Strawberry smoothie – add ¼ cup strawberries for a pink delight that will please even the fussiest of eaters.
- Blueberry smoothie - add 1/3 cup blueberries. Blend thoroughly.
- Banana smoothie – the ultimate filling smoothie! Add mashed banana with cinnamon or simply chop a whole banana into the smoothie and whiz it up.
- Mango and coconut - Add ½ mango and replace the milk with a small tin of coconut milk and water to make ¾ cup.
- Choccie - Add a spoonful of cocoa and half an avocado for a choccie hit that is packed with green goodness. Go on try it, it is yummier than it sounds! OR try a chocolate protein powder instead of the cocoa. This will mix beautifully with either strawberries or a banana.

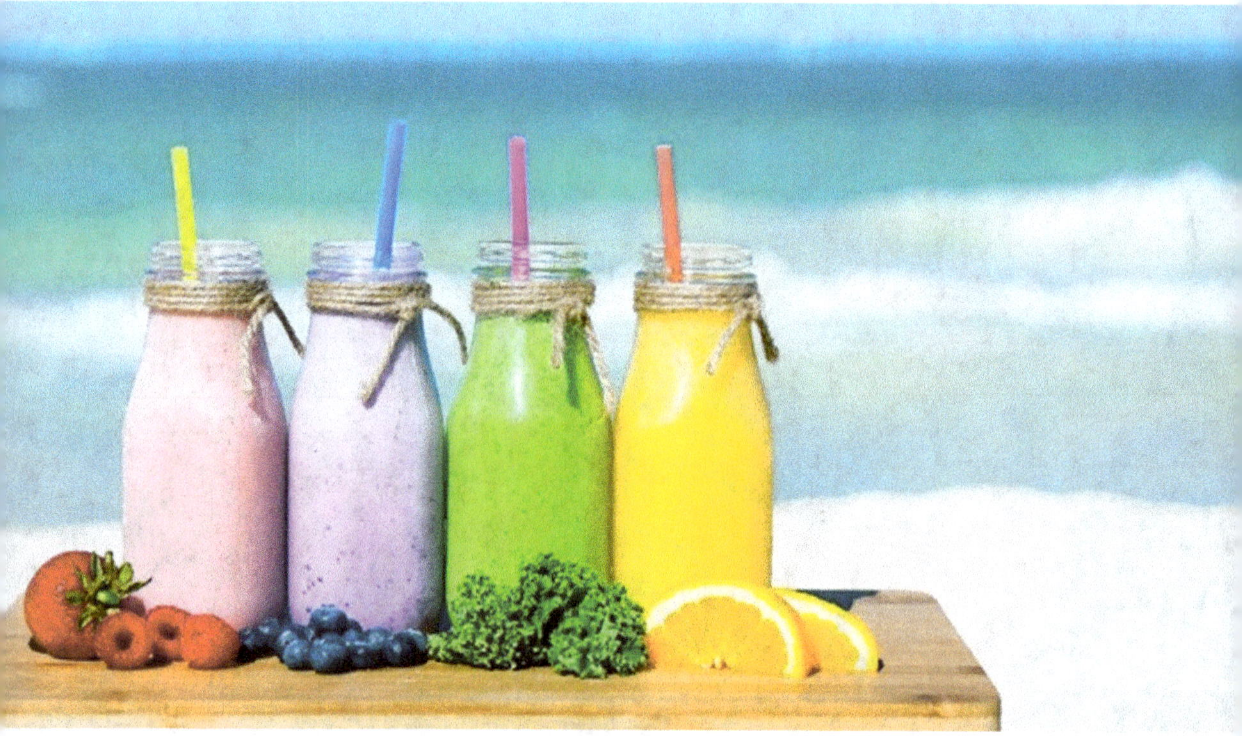

SOFT FOOD IDEAS *for* DINNER

Scrambled Eggs - a great protein source

Ingredients
- 15g butter
- 6 eggs, lightly beaten
- 1/3 cup cooking cream

Method
1. Crack the eggs into a mixing bowl and add the cream, salt and pepper and whisk until combined.
2. Melt the butter in a frying pan on a medium heat and swirl the melted butter to evenly coat the base of the pan.
3. Tip the egg mix into the pan and let it sit for 30 seconds, then gently fold the mixture from the outside in for a further 2 minutes.
4. Serve scrambled eggs on top of soft bread cut into soldiers.

Tip: Add 100g of chopped smoked salmon to the pan halfway thru cooking the eggs.

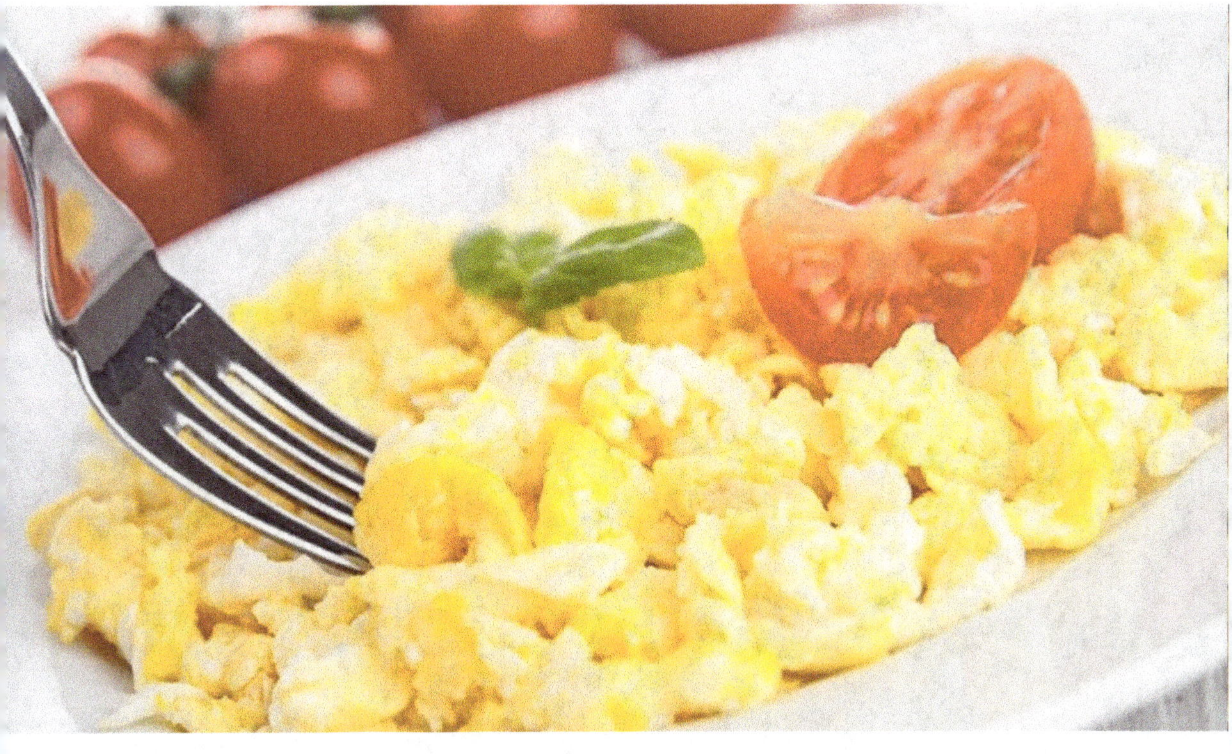

SOFT FOOD IDEAS *for* DINNER

Tofu Scramble - great for vegetarians/vegans

This is a great alternative to scrambled eggs and is suitable for vegans.

Ingredients
- 280g block of tofu
- ½ tsp smoked paprika
- 1 tsp ground cumin
- 1 tbsp olive oil
- Salt and pepper

Method
1. Mash the tofu using a fork.
2. Heat the oil in a frypan and fry the mashed tofu on a medium heat for a few minutes.
3. Sprinkle with paprika and cumin and cook for a few more minutes, constantly stirring and lipping to ensure the tofu does not catch.
4. Season with salt & pepper. Serve with soft bread or a side of fresh chopped avocado.

Variation: Add finely diced, deseeded tomatoes & handful of mushrooms cut in small pieces.

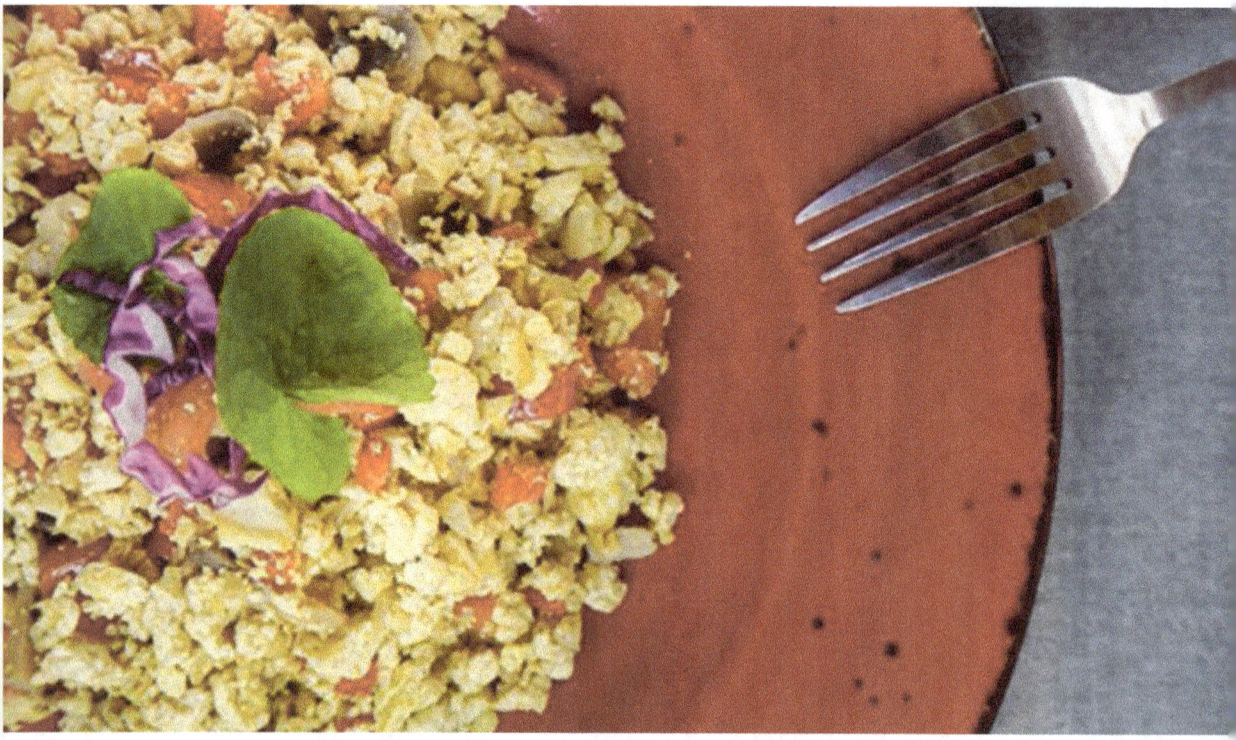

SOFT FOOD IDEAS *for* DINNER

Pancakes - a family favourite

Ingredients
- 1 cup plain flour
- 2 tbsp caster sugar
- 1 egg
- ½ tsp vanilla essence
- 1 cup milk
- Canola oil for cooking Maple syrup (optional)

Method
1. Sift flour into a bowl, add the sugar and mix.
2. Whisk ¾ cup milk, egg and vanilla together then add to the lour and mix well.
3. Add the remaining milk if needed to make a thick consistency.
4. Melt 1 tbsp butter in a frypan on medium heat and spread evenly.
5. Add a soup ladle of mixture to the pan.
6. When bubbles appear, lip using a spatula and cook the other side until lightly browned.
7. Serve with chopped banana or mango and a drizzle of maple syrup.

Serving Idea: Serve with chopped banana or mango and a drizzle of maple syrup.
Variation Idea: This recipe is for thinner style pancakes. If you want thicker pancakes, swap the plain flour for self-raising flour.

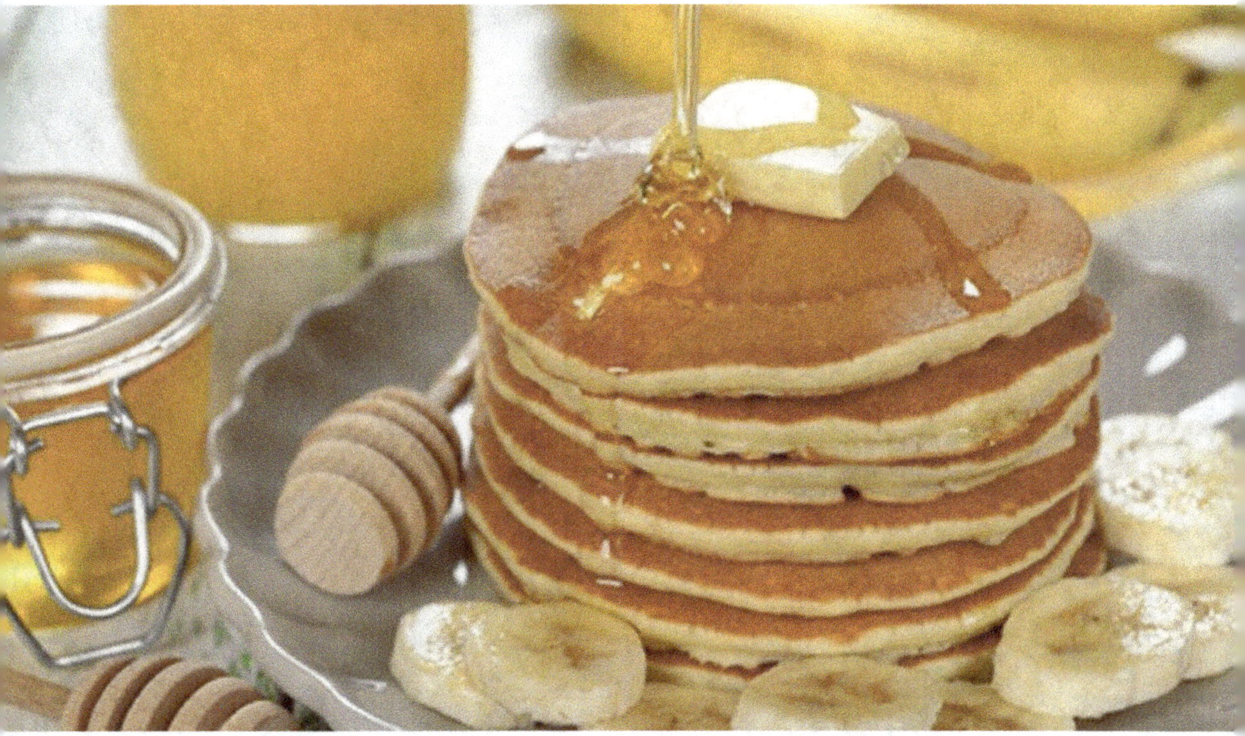

SOFT FOOD IDEAS *for* DINNER

Pikelets - brilliant snacks and lunch box fillers

About this Recipe: these are one of the first things I learnt to cook by myself and have become a lifelong favourite. For many years I left the egg out to make egg-free and also substituted the milk for rice milk. They still turn out delicious but do burn easily so need to be watched carefully.

Ingredients
- 1 ½ cups SR Flour
- 3 tbs raw sugar
- 1 egg
- 1 cup milk

Method
1. Sift flour into a bowl, add the sugar and mix.
2. Whisk ¾ cup milk and the egg together then add to the flour and mix well.
3. Add the remaining milk if needed to make a thick consistency.
4. Melt 1 tbsp butter in a frypan on medium heat and spread evenly.
5. Add dessertspoons of mixture and watch as they start to bubble.
6. When bubbles appear, flip using a spatula and cook the other side until lightly browned.

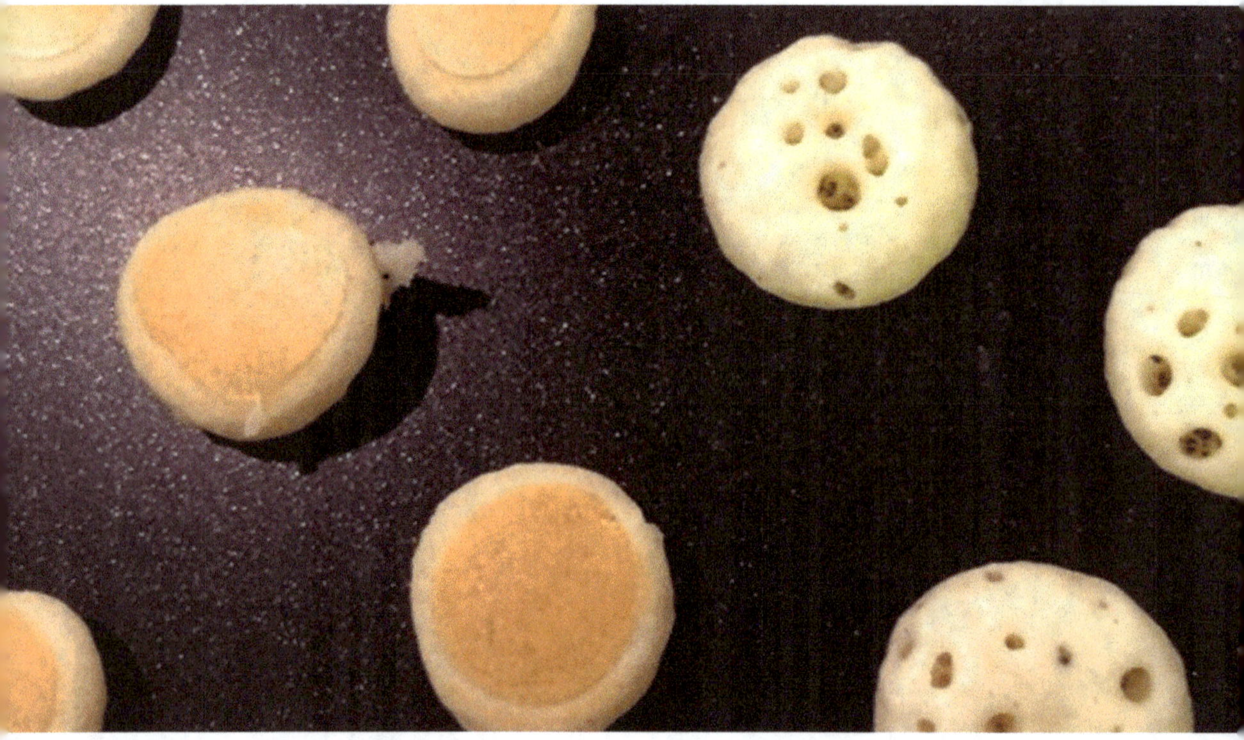

SOFT FOOD IDEAS *for* DINNER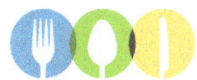

Creamy Mushroom Open Sandwich - Yum!

Ingredients
- 1 or 2 Slices of Sourdough (crusts removed) or any soft bread
- 100g mushrooms sliced
- 3 tbsp sour cream (optional) Salt and pepper
- 2 tbsp butter for cooking

Method
1. Melt butter in a frypan on medium heat.
2. Add the mushrooms and move around the pan until lightly browned and soft.
3. If using sour cream, add to the pan and stir until just mixed.
4. Season with salt and pepper.
5. Serve immediately on a slice of soft bread with crusts removed.

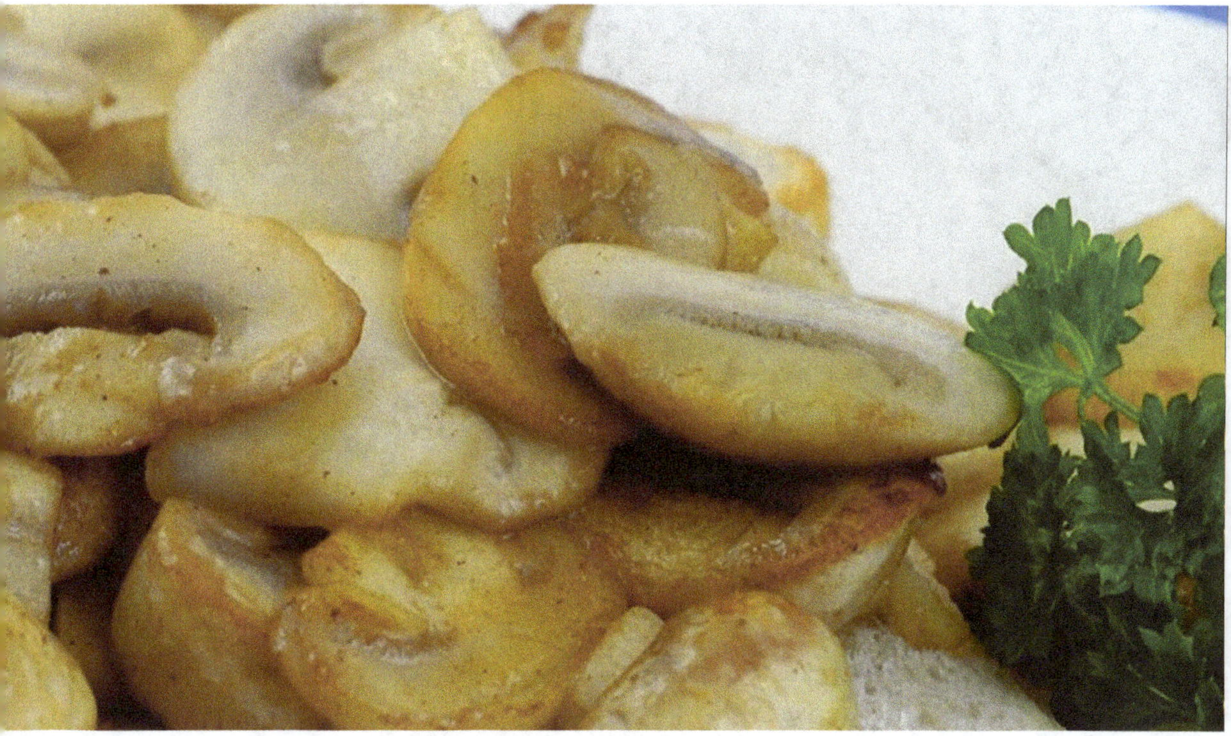

SOFT FOOD IDEAS for DINNER

Muffins – the perfect brunch or lunchbox food

Muffins have always been a firm favourite in our house. Great for snacks, breakfast and such a great option for lunchboxes. For many years we have made ours without eggs and they turn out perfectly fine. In recent years we have started to add an egg and found that this does help them last a bit longer as they are not as dry. However, if you or anyone in your house is allergic to eggs, just leave the eggs out!

Pear and Dark Chocolate Muffins -crowd-pleaser!

Ingredients
- 2 cups SR Flour
- ½ cup caster sugar
- ¼ cup melted butter
- 300ml milk (any type of milk can be used – cow's, almond, rice milk)
- 1 egg (optional)
- 2 x 120g store-bought diced pears in juice 150g Dark choc chips
- ½ tsp vanilla extract

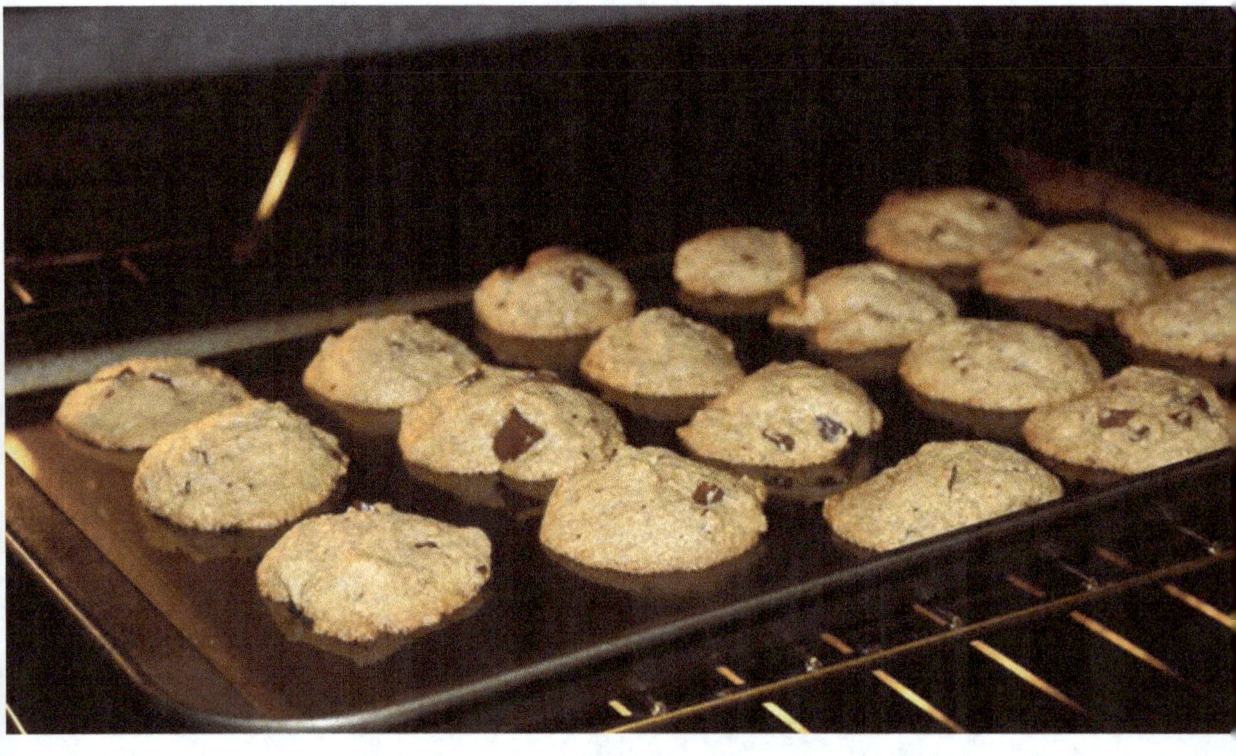

SOFT FOOD IDEAS *for* DINNER

Method

1. Pre-heat the oven to 200 degrees Celsius and Line a muffin tray with patty pans.
2. Combine flour and sugar in a bowl.
3. Melt the butter in the microwave in 20 second bursts until just melted.
4. Make a well in the four and sugar mix.
5. Tip in the milk, butter and vanilla, mix lightly.
6. Whisk the egg in a small bowl and then add to the large bowl.
7. Mix lightly then add the pears and dark chocolate chips.
8. Mix until just combined and chunky ingredients are mixed in.
9. Bake for 15 to 20 minutes or until a skewer comes out clean when inserted into the middle of a muffin.

Variations:
- Apple and sultana muffins: swap the chopped pears and dark chocolate chips for chopped cooked apples and 100g sultanas (the sultanas will go soft).
- Double Chocolate: add 1.5 tablespoons of cocoa powder, leave out the fruit and add 50g white chocolate chips for a chocolate extravaganza!

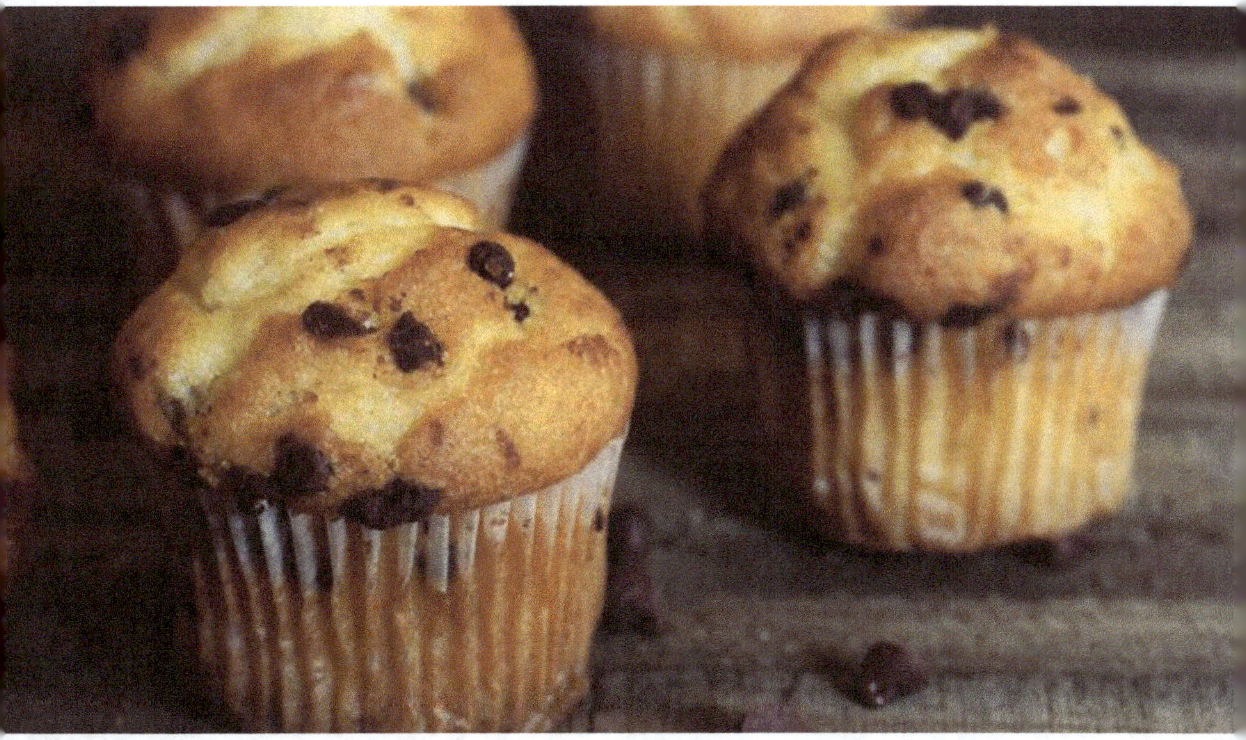

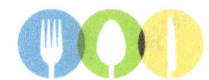

SOFT FOOD IDEAS *for* DINNER

Lunch and Dinner Recipes

This section starts off with light meals and moves on to more substantial recipes. The light meals are great for when your teeth and gums and sore and are also terrific side dishes to have with some of the substantial and meatier meals.

Mashed potatoes - your secret weapon

Mashed potatoes are your secret weapon! Why? Well, it is filling. It is non-acidic so perfect for when you have sore gums or ulcers. It is plain and so soft that you do not need to use your teeth at all. Best of all, even the fussiest of eaters likes potatoes! All these reasons make the humble mash one of your best go-to foods for sore teeth and sensitive gums.

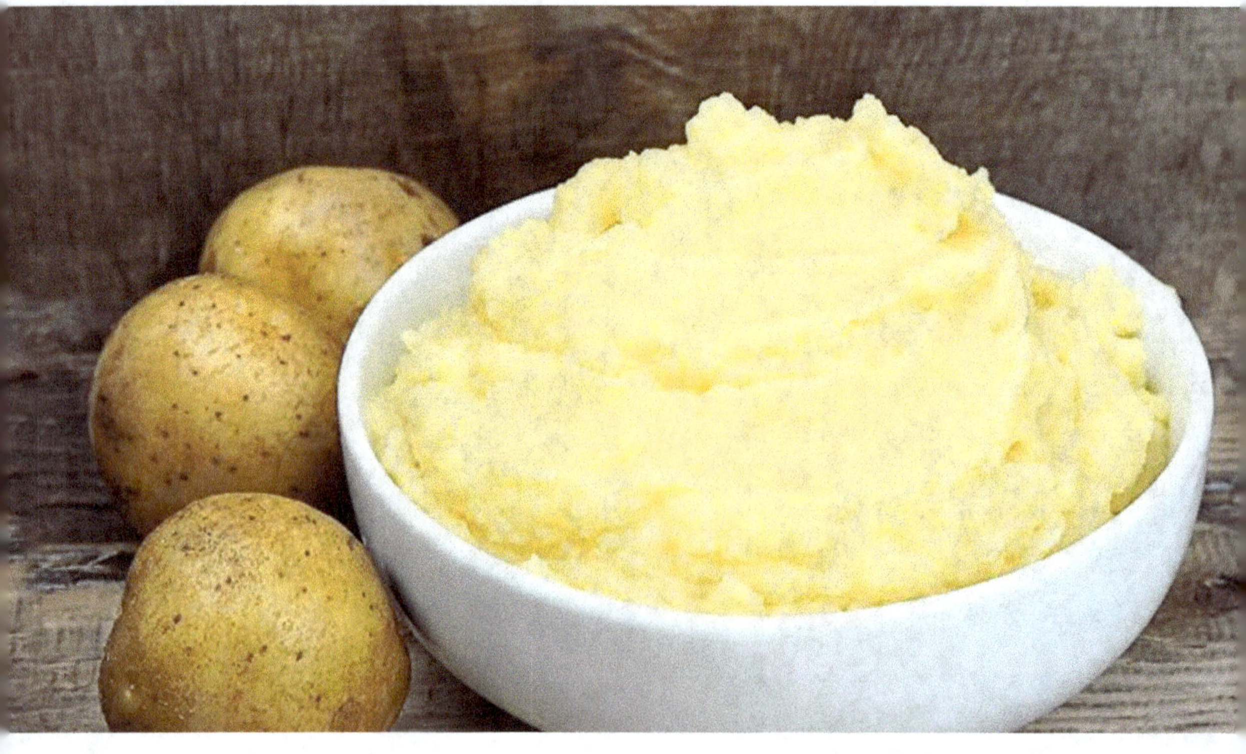

SOFT FOOD IDEAS *for* DINNER

Guacamole – Good Old Smashed Avo!

Ingredients
- 1 Avocado, halved, stone removed, fresh chopped and peeled
- ½ Tomato, seeds and pulp discarded, fresh finely chopped (optional)
- Salt and pepper

Method
1. Place the chopped avocado in a bowl and mash with a fork.
2. Fold in diced tomato
3. Season with salt and pepper.
4. Serve on soft bread (with crust removed).

Tip: Most guacamole recipes use lime juice which I have omitted here as the acidity of the citrus can sting on sore gums.

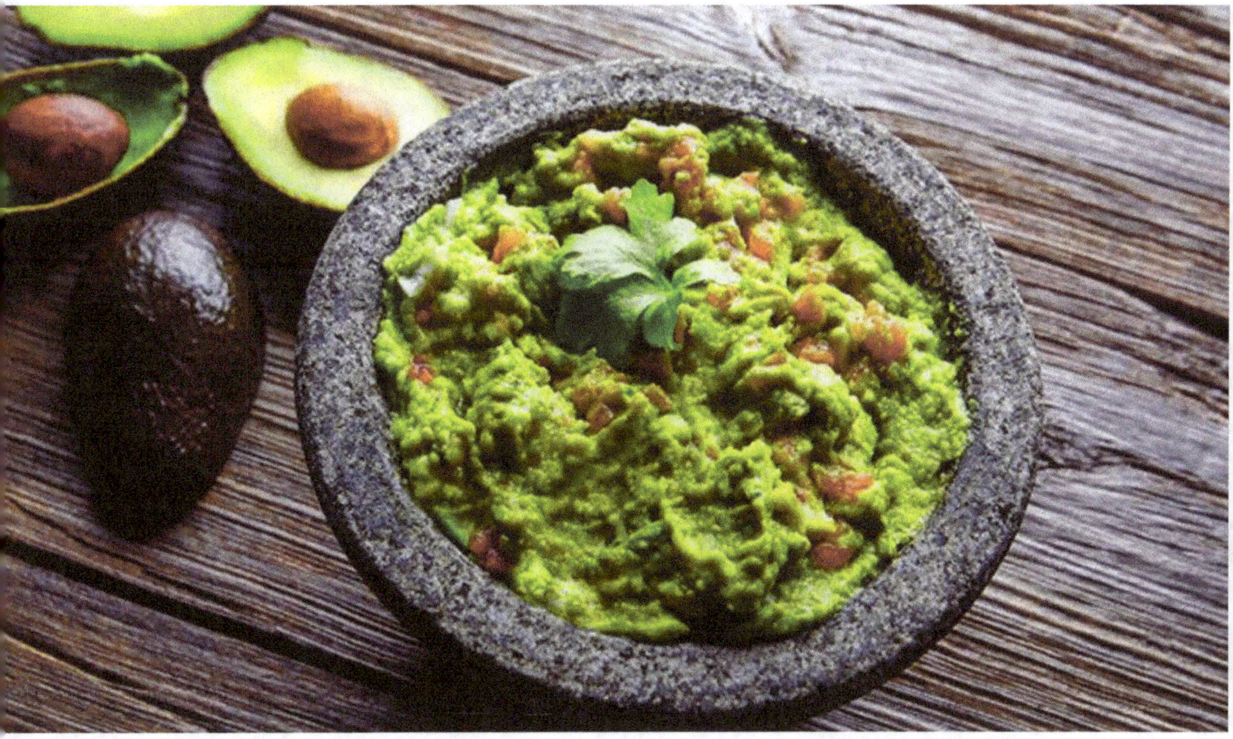

# SOFT FOOD IDEAS *for* DINNER

Potato Salad – brilliant side dish or lunch box filler

Ingredients
- 1kg White potatoes
- ½ cup mayonnaise
- ½ cup sour cream
- 1 tsp Dijon mustard
- 100g lunch meat – ham or turkey – cut into ribbons
- Herbs of choice (optional)

Method
1. Peel and dice potatoes into 1 inch cubes.
2. Boil a large pot of salted water.
3. Add potatoes and cook for 10 minutes or until potatoes are just cooked.
4. Strain potatoes in a colander and allow to cool.
5. Mix mayo, sour cream and mustard then season with salt and pepper.
6. Toss the creamy mix with the potatoes and meat in a large bowl.
7. Add herbs such as finely chopped parsley or chives but if these small pieces are a problem, just leave them out.

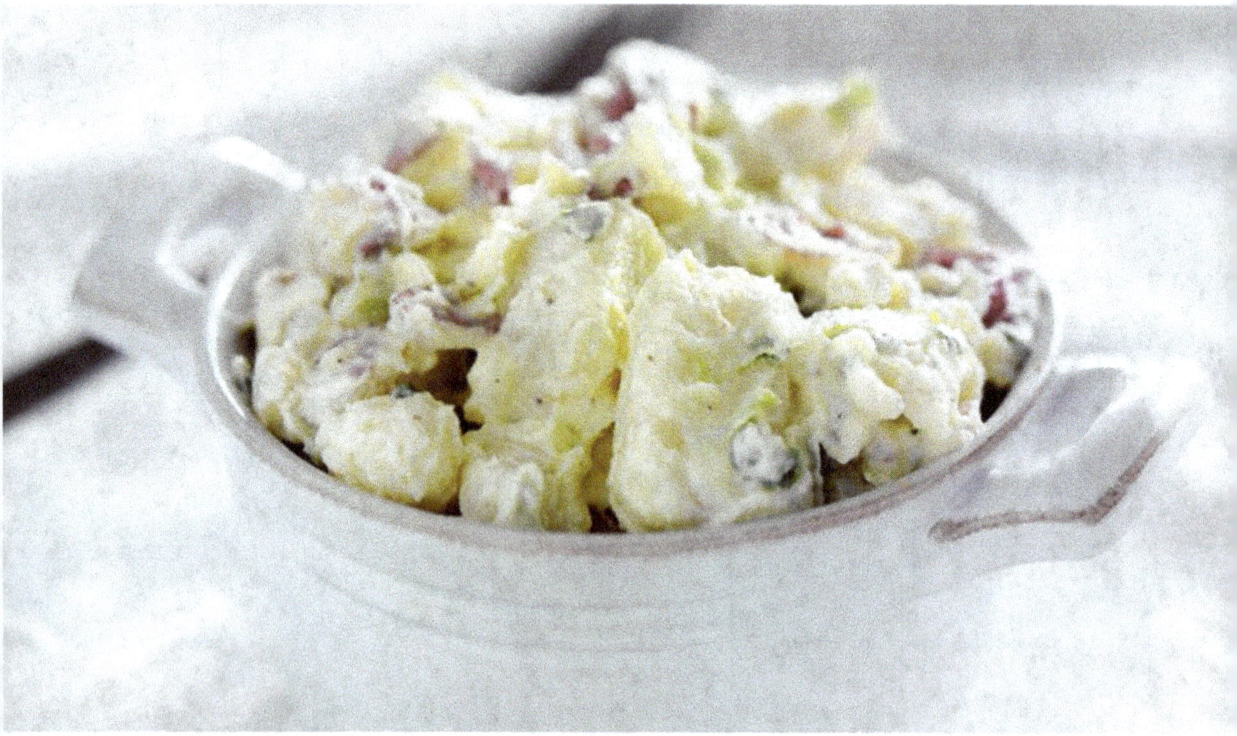

SOFT FOOD IDEAS *for* DINNER

Lettuce and Blue Cheese salad - tasty lunch or side dish

Ingredients
- ¼ Iceberg lettuce, shredded
- 1 eating apple cut into matchsticks
- 8 thin slices of cucumber cut into quarters
- 20g Blue Cheese
- Honey to drizzle

Method
1. Shred the lettuce and chop the cucumber and apple into thin slices or matchsticks.
2. Place the lettuce in a bowl, top with the apple and cucumber, and crumble the blue cheese over the top.
3. Drizzle with honey then serve.

Ideas:
- If you don't like blue cheese, substitute with your cheese of choice, just be sure to avoid hard cheeses.
- Top with any herbs you may have on hand. Chives or dill would be lovely. You can also put this combination in a wrap and add mayo.
- Add a small tin of tuna or salmon and turn into a substantial meal.

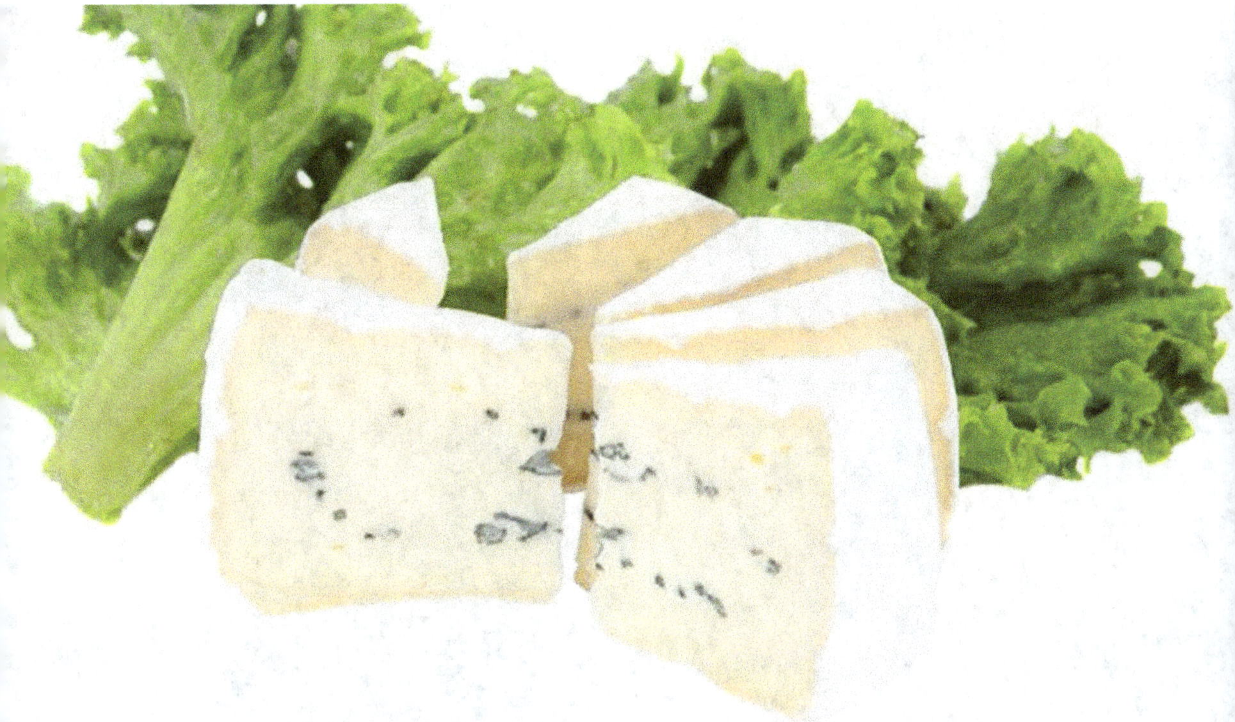

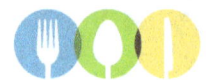

SOFT FOOD IDEAS for DINNER

Fish Patties - simply delicious

Ingredients
- 750g raw white fish fillets
- ¼ breadcrumbs
- ½ brown onion grated
- 1 tsp lemon zest
- ¼ cup dill or parsley finely chopped
- 1 egg*
- Salt and pepper
- Vegetable oil for cooking

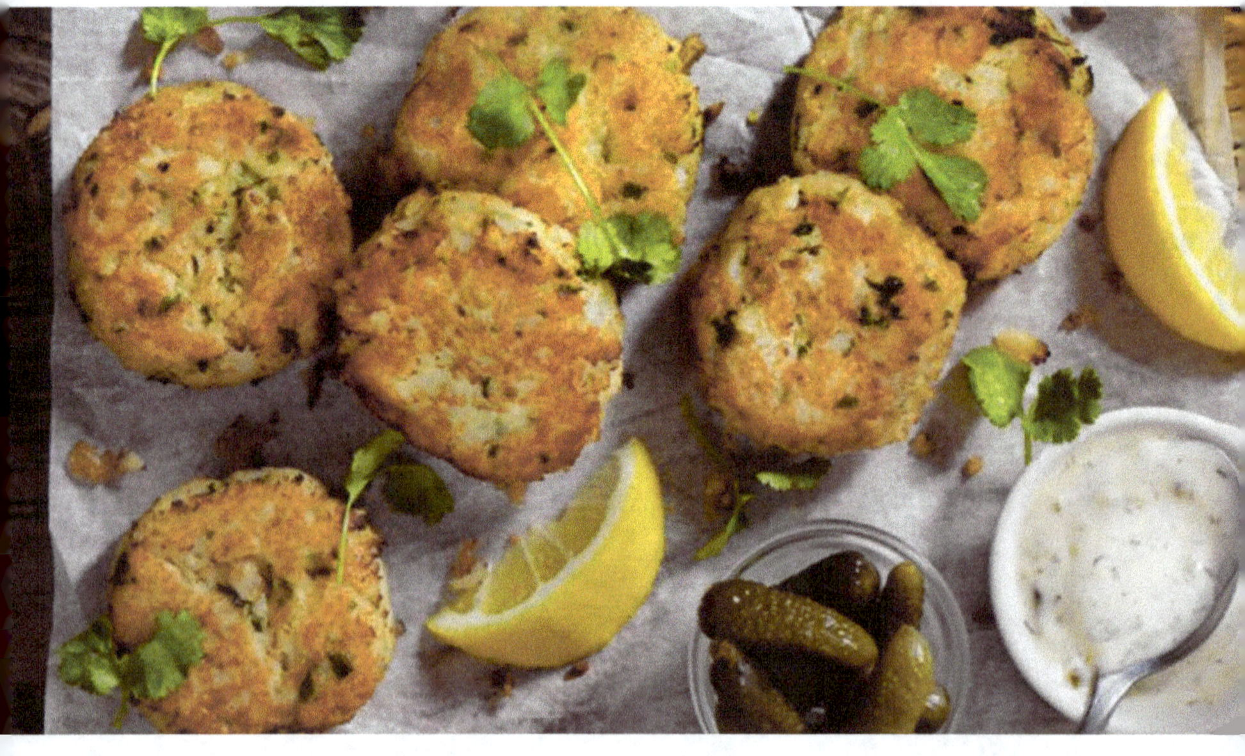

SOFT FOOD IDEAS *for* DINNER

Ingredients
- 750g raw white fish fillets
- ¼ breadcrumbs
- ½ brown onion grated
- 1 tsp lemon zest
- ¼ cup dill or parsley finely chopped
- 1 egg*
- Salt and pepper
- Vegetable oil for cooking

Method
1. Roughly chop fish and put into a food processor. Pulse until chopped, be careful not to overwork the fish or it will turn into a paste.
2. Put fish, breadcrumbs, onion, lemon zest, herbs and egg in a bowl and mix together.
3. Season well with salt and pepper.
4. Add a tablespoon of oil to a frypan on a moderate heat.
5. Use a tablespoon to scoop the fish mixture and add to the pan, pressing the fish cake gently with the back of the spoon to even out.
6. Cook for a couple of minutes on each side.
7. Repeat in batches until all mixture has been used.
8. Eat on their own with mayo or tartare sauce or make it a more substantial meal by serving with mashed potatoes.

Variation Idea:
To make this egg free, add 2 tablespoons of plain flour. This will help bind the mixture. Swap the white fish for two 415g tins of Red or Pink Salmon. Instead of step 1 above, do this: Open the tins, drain and remove excess skin and bones. Then use your hands to lake the salmon into the mixing bowl and mix together with the other ingredients.

SOFT FOOD IDEAS *for* DINNER

Potato and Leek Soup - smooth and satisfying

This is the perfect first week meal. Everyone loves potatoes and it is a quite easy soup to make. Best of all, it will please even the fussiest of eaters.

Ingredients
- 8 medium size white potatoes
- 1 Leek thinly sliced
- 1 litre Chicken Stock
- 1 tbsp Olive Oil
- 2 tbsp Cooking Cream (optional)
- Salt and White Pepper

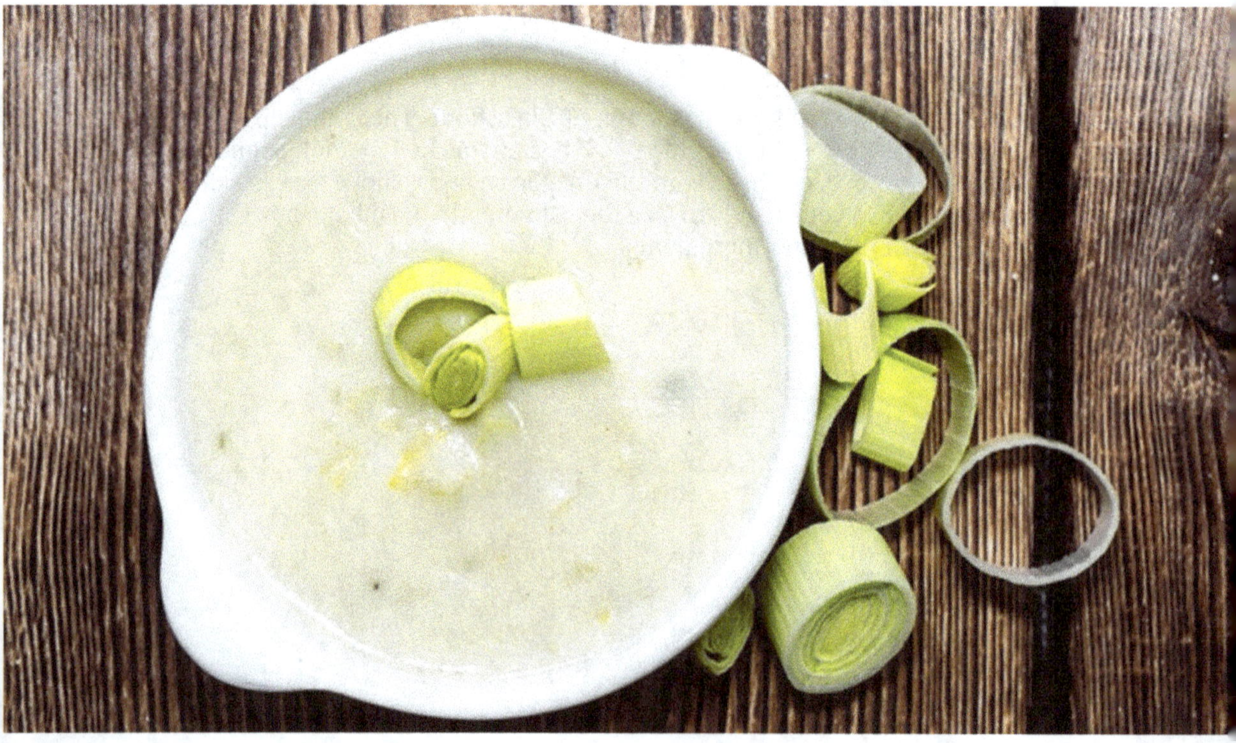

SOFT FOOD IDEAS *for* DINNER

Method
1. Thinly sliced the white part of the leek.
2. Heat the olive oil in a large pot then add the leek and cook until soft but not brown.
3. Peel and roughly chop the potatoes then add to the pan along with the chicken stock.
4. Bring to the boil then simmer for 15 minutes or until the potatoes are soft.
5. Take off the heat and use a stab mixer to puree until smooth.
6. Add the cream and add small amounts of water to thin out soup if necessary.
7. Season with salt and white pepper.

Serving Idea:
Serve with soft white bread (no seeds!) such as Brioche– or - use any non-seeded bread, cut the hard crusts off (use these to make breadcrumbs and freeze), and cut into small cubes and sprinkle on top of the soup. The fresh bread 'croutons will soak up the soup and be nice and soft to eat. This will help make the soup feel more filling.

SOFT FOOD IDEAS for DINNER

Fish Chowder - so tasty!

Ingredients
- 50g butter
- 1 leek finely sliced
- 1 carrot diced into 1cm cubes
- 1 celery stalk finely chopped
- 2 potatoes, peeled and diced into 1 cm pieces
- 1 tbsp cornflour
- 3 cups fish or chicken stock
- 500 g white fish fillet chopped
- ½ cup cream
- Salt and pepper

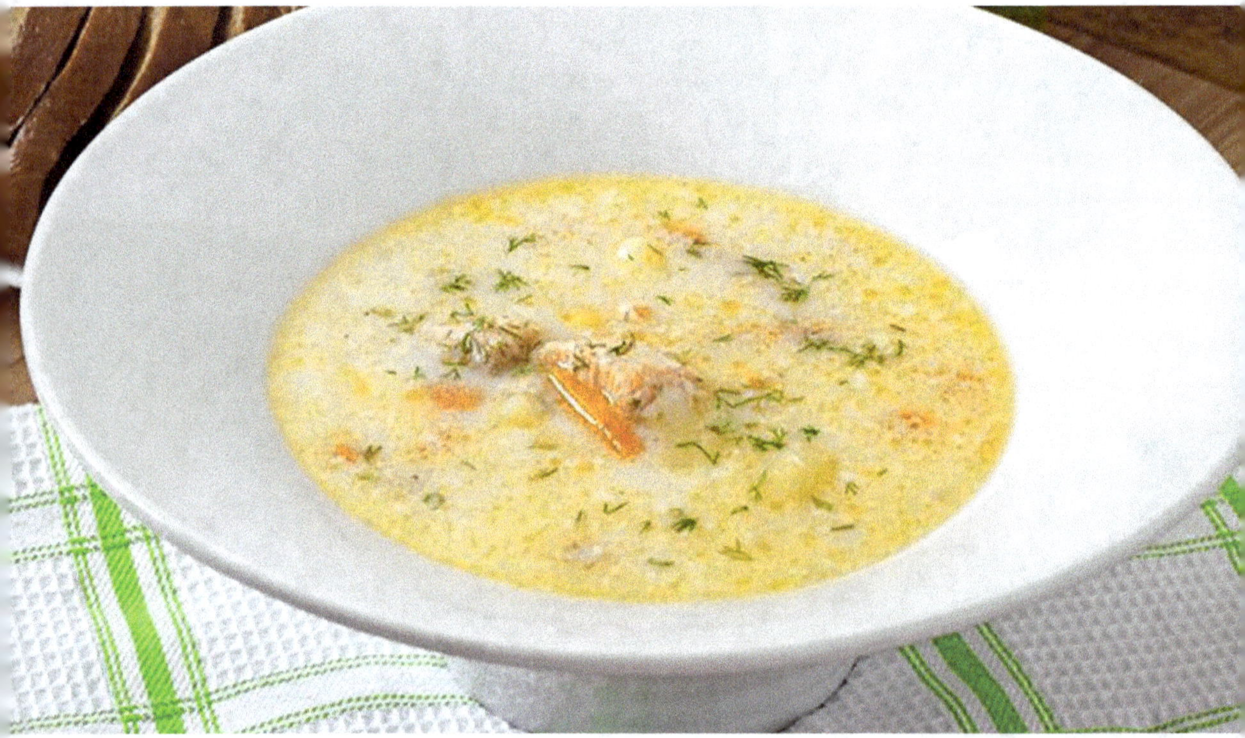

SOFT FOOD IDEAS *for* DINNER

Method
1. Melt a tablespoon of the butter then add the leek, carrot, celery and potatoes.
2. Cook over a moderate heat, stirring to prevent the vegetables catching on the pan, until the carrot has just softened. Don't worry if the potatoes are not cooked thru at this stage.
3. Push the vegetables to one side of the pan and add the remaining butter. When melted add the cornflour and mix to make a roux.
4. Add the stock one ladle full at a time and vigourously mix with the roux to ensure no lumps. Keep adding the remaining stock and mix with the vegetables.
5. Bring to the boil, then lower the heat and simmer for a few minutes. The potatoes should now be soft, and the mixture has slightly thickened.
6. Using a stab mixer, puree half of the soup so that it is half chunky and half pureed.
7. Add the fish and cook for a few more minutes until it is cooked thru.
8. If you would prefer a smoother chowder, use the stab mixer again and puree your soup to the desired consistency.
9. Add the cream, heat thru without bringing to the boil.
10. If the soup is a little thick, add soup ladles of stock one at a time and mix until the desired consistency is reached.
11. Season with salt and pepper and your soup is ready.

Serving Idea:
Serve with some soft brioche or chop up any type of bread into cubes and place on top to soften and help fill you up!

SOFT FOOD IDEAS for DINNER

Corn Chowder - great comfort food

Ingredients
- 50g butter
- 1 onion finely sliced
- 1 carrot diced into 1cm cubes
- 1 celery stalk finely chopped
- 1 potato, peeled and diced into 1 cm pieces
- 3 cups fish, vegetable or chicken stock 500g frozen corn kernels
- ½ cup cream
- Salt and pepper

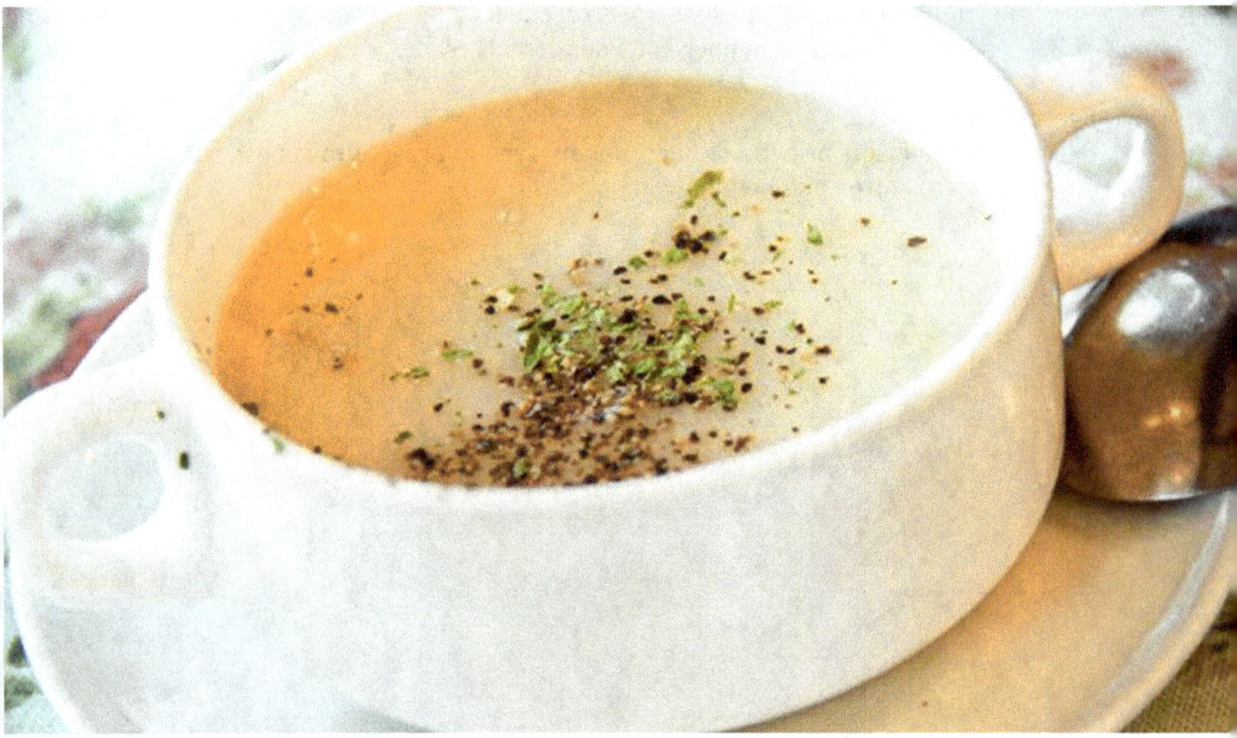

SOFT FOOD IDEAS *for* DINNER

Method
1. Melt a tablespoon of the butter then add the onion, carrot, celery and potato.
2. Cook over a moderate heat, stirring to prevent the vegetables catching on the pan, until the vegetables have softened and lightly browned.
3. Add the stock and corn kernels and bring to the boil, then lower the heat and simmer for a few minutes.
4. Add the cream, heat thru without bringing to the boil.
5. Using a stab mixer, puree the soup. Puree until completely smooth.
6. If the soup is a little thick, add additional ladles of stock until the desired consistency is reached.
7. Season with salt and pepper and your soup is ready.

Serving Idea:
Serve with some soft brioche or chop up any type of bread into cubes and place on top to soften and help fill you up!

SOFT FOOD IDEAS for DINNER

Chicken Noodle Soup - Soul food!

Ingredients
- 2 tbsp olive oil
- 1 brown onion, finely chopped
- 1 medium carrot, peeled and sliced thinly
- 1 stick celery, finely diced
- 1 medium potato, peeled and diced into 1cm pieces
- 3 cups chicken stock
- 1 store-bought BBQ chicken or 250g (approx.) chicken breast fillet
- 100g rice noodles or small pasta shapes
- 1/2 tsp mild curry powder

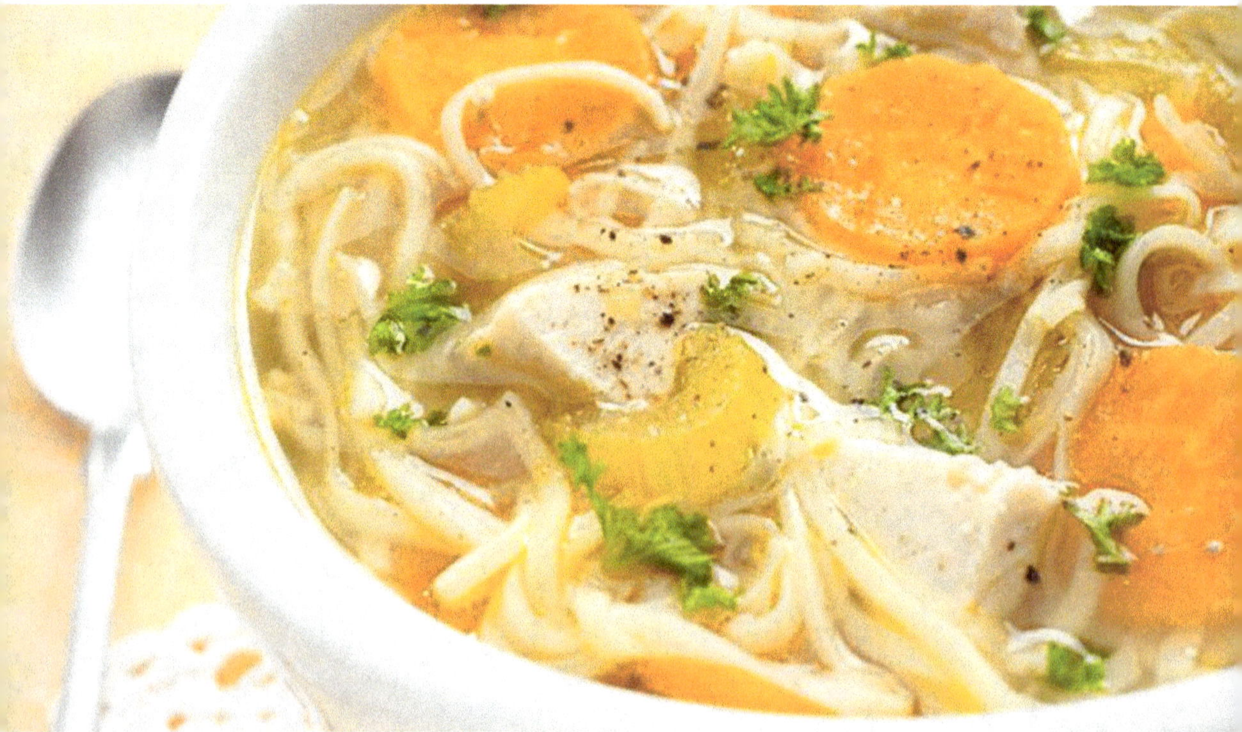

SOFT FOOD IDEAS *for* DINNER

Method
1. Heat oil in pan, add curry powder (it is only a small amount but makes a big difference), onion, carrot, celery and potato and cook for 5 to 8 minutes or until vegetables have softened.
2. Add the chicken stock and bring to the boil before reducing heat and simmering for 5 minutes.
3. Remove the breast meat from the chicken and chop into 1cm pieces. Alternately, chop the raw chicken fillet and add to the pan.
4. Use scissors to cut the rice noodles into approximately 1 inch size lengths and add to the pan.
5. Bring to the boil then reduce heat and simmer for 5 to 10 minutes or until the noodles have softened and if using raw meat, that the chicken has cooked thru.
6. Season with salt and pepper and serve with soft bread.

SOFT FOOD IDEAS *for* DINNER

Baked Salmon with steamed vegies

Ingredients
- 4 x skin-free Salmon fillets (or one for each person)
- 2 lemons sliced
- Salt and pepper
- Bunch of asparagus (or any greens you prefer)
- 5 white potatoes peeled and cut into 2 inch pieces
- 1 tbsp olive oil
- 1 tbsp butter

Method
1. Preheat the oven to 200 degrees Celsius.
2. Grease an oven tray and lay the lemon slices out to make a bed.
3. Season the salmon fillets with sea salt, black pepper and olive oil.
4. Place the salmon fillets on top of the lemon and put in the oven to bake for 12 minutes or until done.
5. Boil the potatoes until tender, then toss with the butter.
6. Boil, steam or pan-fry the asparagus.
7. Serve the salmon with potatoes and asparagus.

Tip: This is equally delicious with any type of white fish and you can swap oven baking for pan-frying.

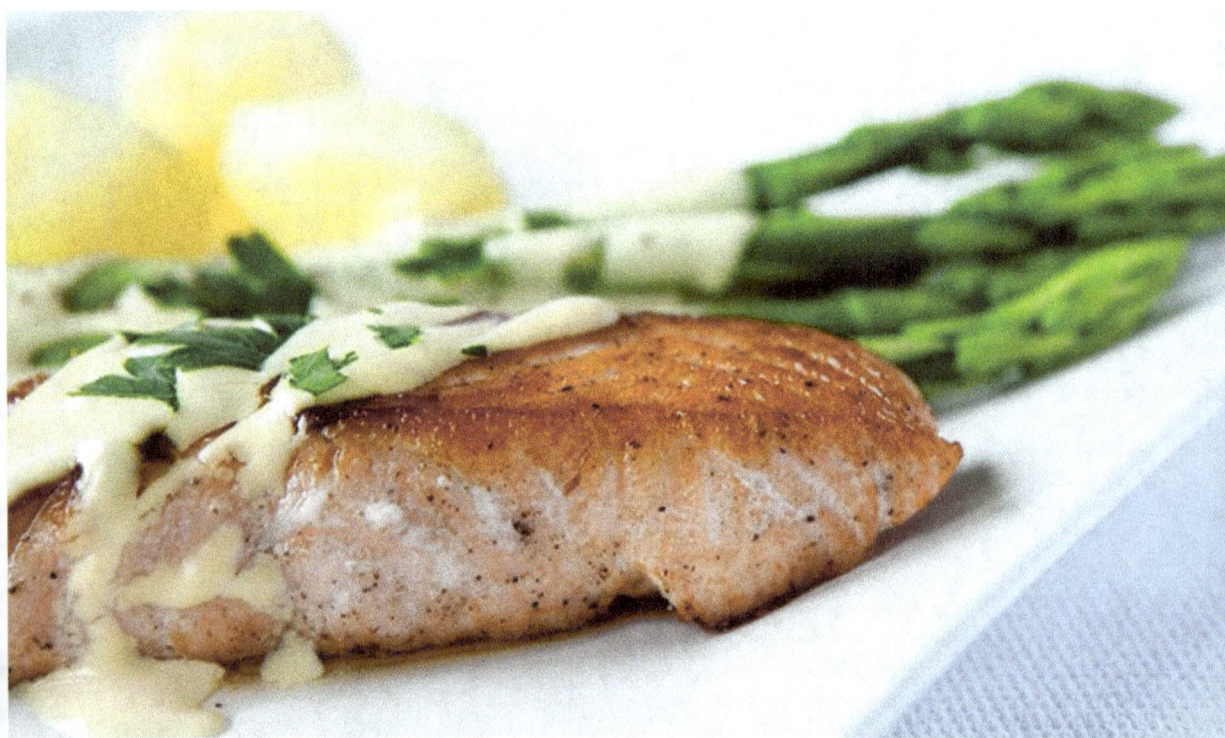

SOFT FOOD IDEAS *for* DINNER

Creamy Salmon and Pea Pasta - a taste sensation!

Ingredients
- 300g macaroni
- 3 tbsp butter
- 1 brown onion, finely diced
- 1 celery stalk, finely diced
- 1 large carrot finely diced
- 2 tbsp cornflour
- 3 cups milk
- 400g raw salmon fillet chopped into 2cm dice or 2 fillets cooked salmon
- 1 cup frozen peas
- 1/3 cup grated parmesan cheese

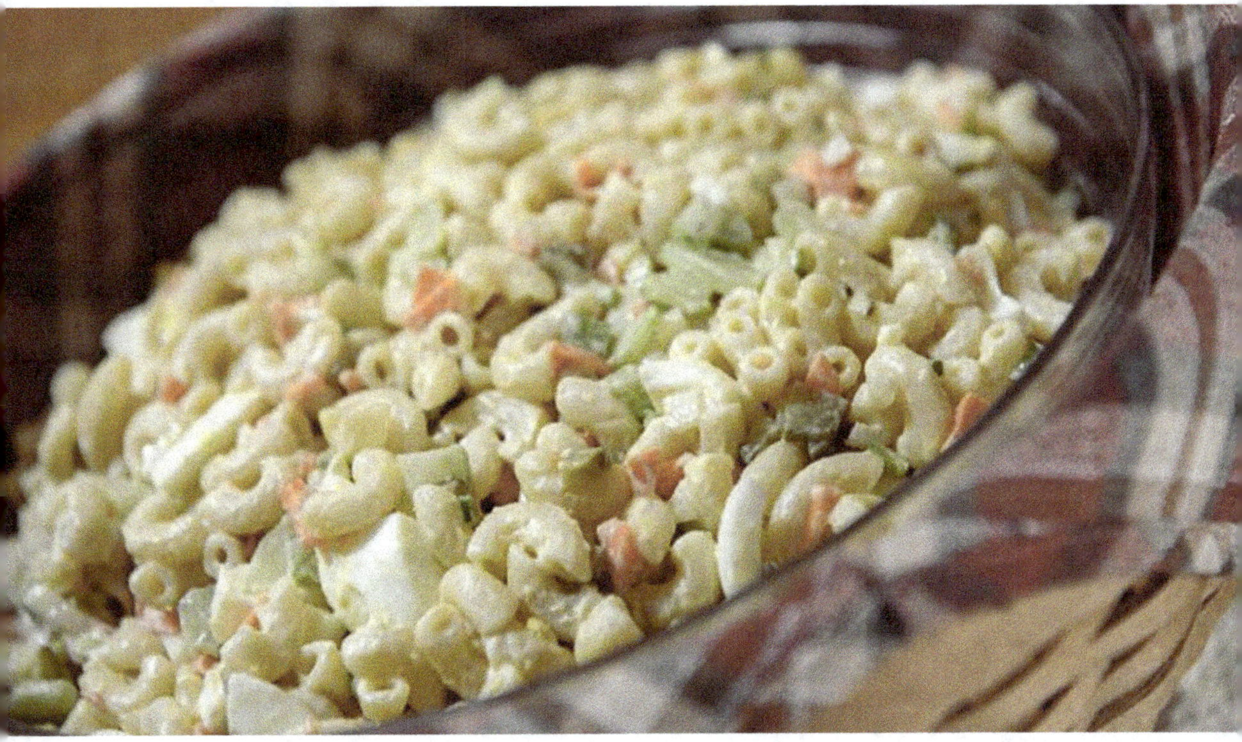

SOFT FOOD IDEAS for DINNER

Method
1. Cook macaroni according to packet directions, drain and put to the side (drizzle with a little olive oil to stop it sticking together).
2. Microwave the peas according to packet directions.
3. Melt 1 tbsp butter in pan and add onion, celery and carrots and stir until softened.
4. Push to one side, add the remaining butter and melt.
5. Add cornflour to the melted butter to make a roux.
6. Gradually add milk, stirring constantly to avoid lumps and start mixing with the vegetables.
7. Once all the milk is added, bring to the boil then reduce heat. Add raw salmon (if using) and cook for 5 minutes. If using hot smoked salmon, add at the end of the 5 minutes.
8. Drain the peas. Add the peas, parmesan and macaroni to the pan and gently combine.
9. Season with pepper and you are ready to serve.

SOFT FOOD IDEAS *for* DINNER

Chicken and Noodle Stir-fry

Ingredients
- 500g chicken mince or chicken thighs cut into small pieces
- 400g noodles – any type of noodles: egg noodles, rice noodles, udon noodles
- 1 carrot cut into sticks
- ½ red capsicum cut into sticks
- ½ cup shredded green cabbage
- 100g bean sprouts
- 2 tbsp Oyster sauce
- 2 tbsp Soy sauce
- 1 tsp pureed ginger (store-bought)

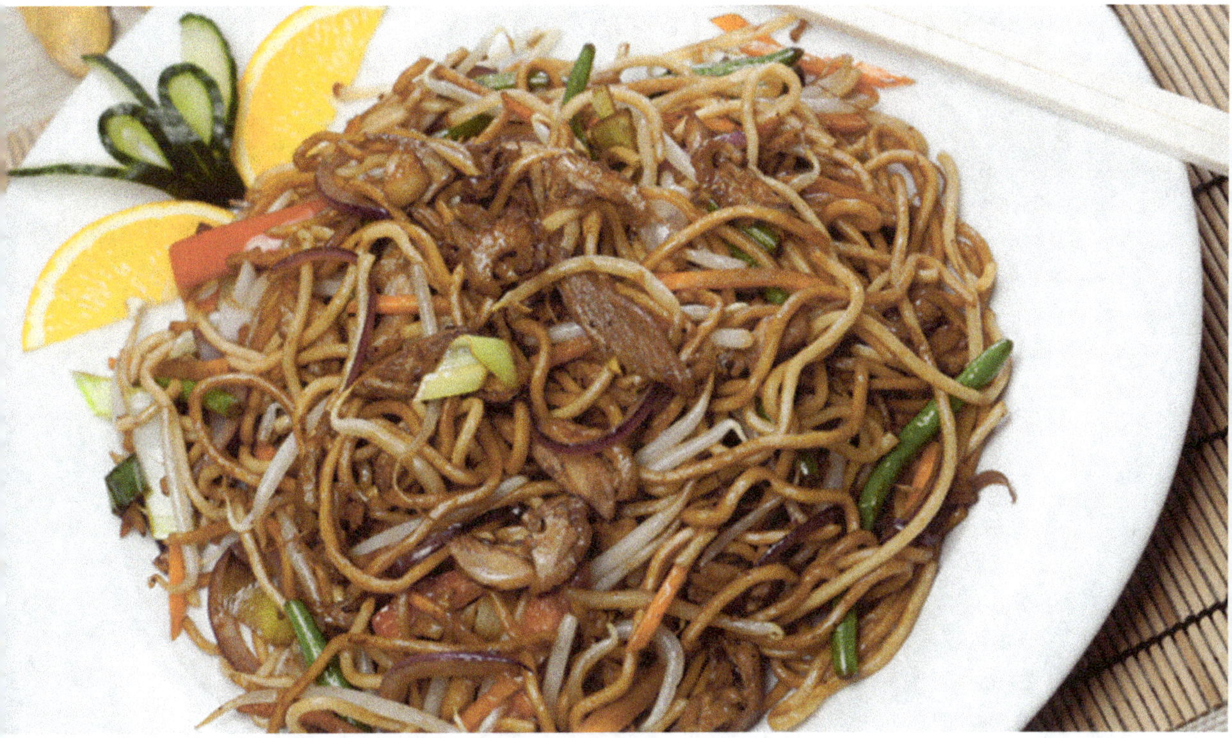

SOFT FOOD IDEAS for DINNER

Method
1. Prepare your chosen noodles as per packet directions and put to one side while preparing everything else.
2. Heat 1 tbsp oil in a wok on high heat.
3. Add the chicken, ginger and tablespoon of soy sauce and stir-fry until the chicken is cooked.
4. Add the carrot, capsicum and cabbage and stir-fry for a few minutes.
5. Add the oyster sauce and remaining tablespoon of soy sauce and stir quickly.
6. Add the bean sprouts and noodles and toss until the noodles are coated in sauce (add a couple of splashes of water if needed).

Variations:
- Add Eggs - After adding the noodles and mixing for a minute, push all ingredients to one side of the wok, then add two whisked eggs to the pan and keep scrambling. When cooked thru, fold the noodle mixture back over the top and mix the eggs thru.
- Any type of meat can be used in this recipe. Substitute the chicken for beef, or even add shrimps.

SOFT FOOD IDEAS *for* DINNER

Meatloaf - great as tasty leftovers in lunchboxes!

Ingredients
- 500g Pork mince
- 1 grated carrot
- 1 minced or grated onion 50g breadcrumbs
- 30g feta cheese
- 1 tablespoon chopped fresh oregano or 1stp dried oregano Sea salt and white pepper
- Olive oil

Method
1. Pre-heat the oven to 200 degrees Celsius.
2. Add the mince, carrot, onion, herbs and breadcrumbs to a bowl.
3. Crumbled in the feta and mix with your hands.
4. Season with salt and pepper.
5. Line a baking tray with baking paper, shape the mixture in a log and place on tray.
6. Drizzle with olive oil, then place in the oven to cook for 20 to 25 minutes or until lightly browned and cooked in the centre.
7. Serve slices of meatloaf with gravy, mashed potatoes or boiled/steamed soft vegetables of your choice.

Tip: Use leftover meatloaf slices as lunch box snacks or for sandwich fillings.

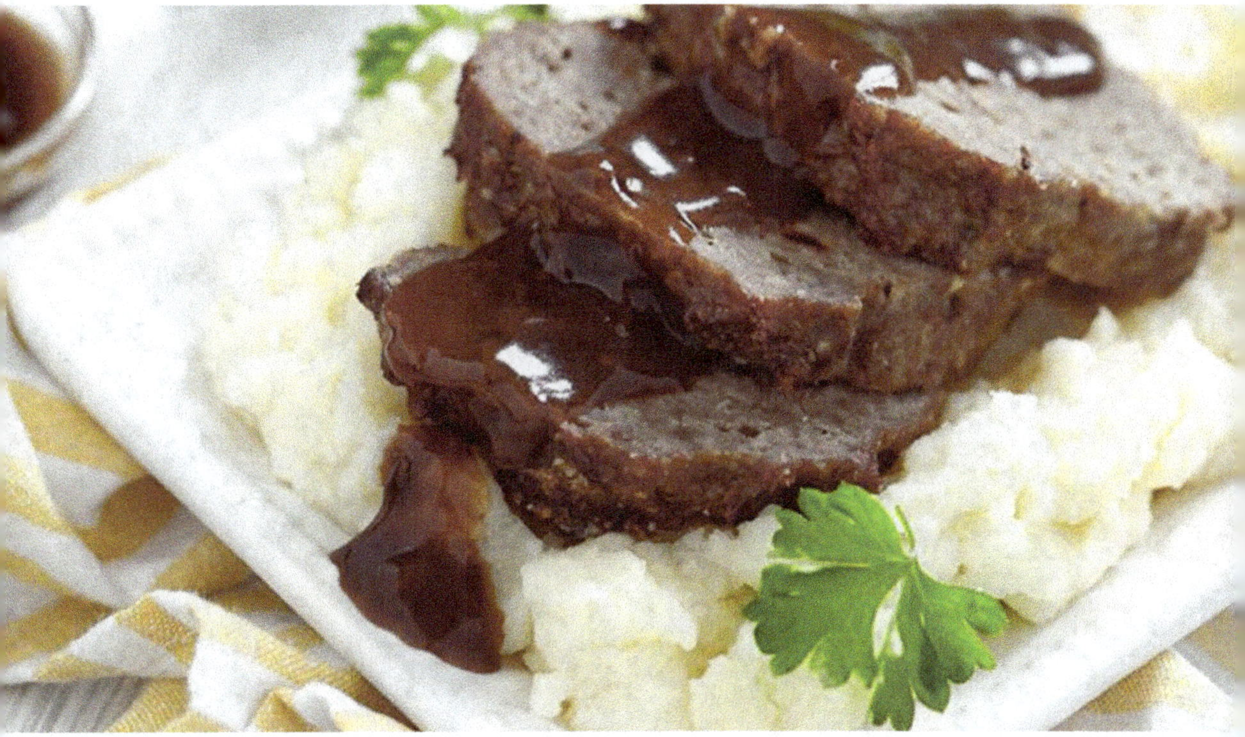

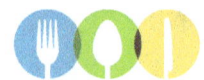

SOFT FOOD IDEAS *for* DINNER

Savoury Mince - a hearty winter warmer

This is a great alternative to Spaghetti Bolognese. The recipe still uses mince so it is easy to eat, but without the staining issues that can be caused by rich tomato sauce. Best of all it is nice and tasty.

Ingredients
- 500g mince – beef, pork or chicken
- ½ cup frozen peas
- 1 medium brown onion, finely chopped
- ½ medium carrot, grated or diced
- 1 garlic clove, grated (optional)
- 1 tbsp cornflour
- 1 beef or chicken stock cube
- 1 tbsp Worcestershire sauce
- 1 tbsp olive oil

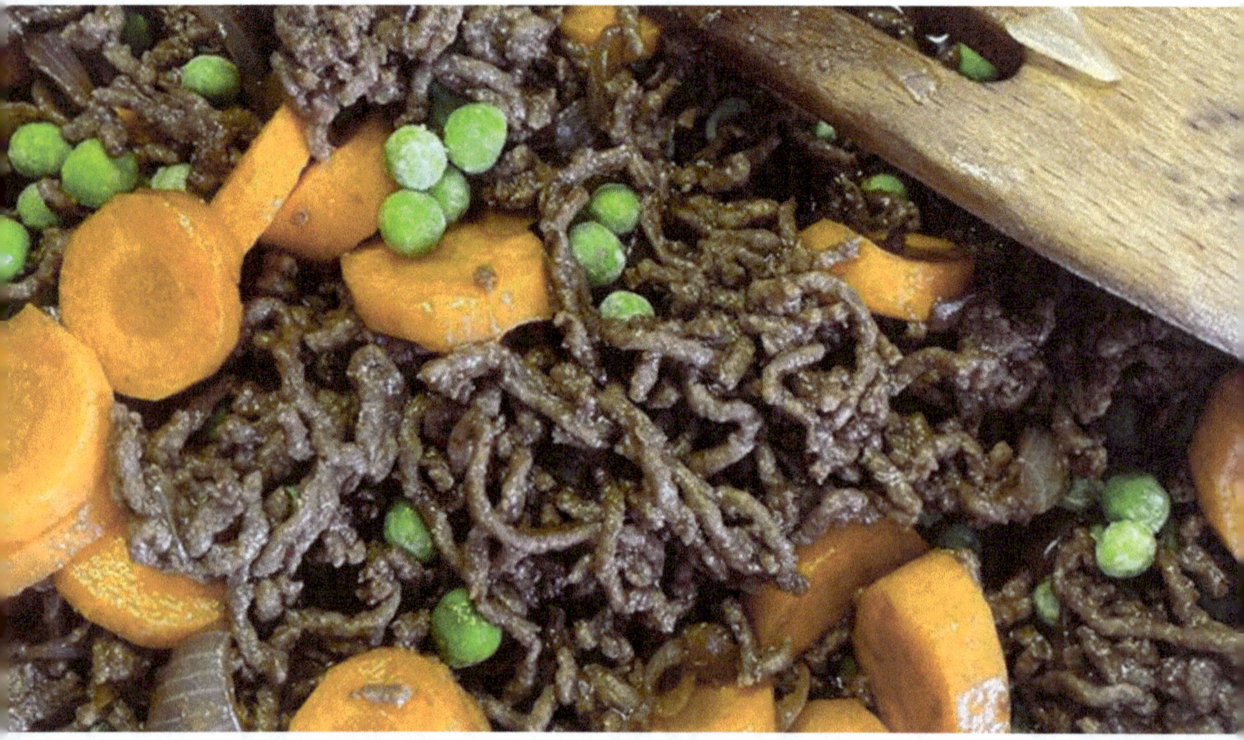

SOFT FOOD IDEAS *for* DINNER

Method
1. Heat oil in a pan over moderate heat.
2. Add carrots and cook for a few minutes before adding the onion and garlic and cook for a further few minutes.
3. Follow the instructions on the packet of peas to cook. My favourite method is to microwave them.
4. Add the mince and break the mince into smaller pieces while stirring.
5. Fill the kettle with water and put on the boil.
6. When the mince has cooked thru and is no longer pink, crumble in the stock cube and add a cup of boiling water from the kettle.
7. Bring to the boil and then reduce to simmer for 10 minutes.
8. Mix the cornflour with 2 tablespoons of water until smooth then add to the mince and stir until thickened.
9. Season with salt and pepper.
10. Add the Worcestershire sauce and peas, stir in for a minute before turning the heat off.

SOFT FOOD IDEAS *for* DINNER

Cottage Pie – classic comfort food

Ingredients
- 1 x Savoury Mince recipe
- 1 x Mashed Potato recipe
- 1 tablespoon grate parmesan

Method
1. Preheat oven to 200 degrees Celsius.
2. Grease a casserole or baking dish.
3. Prepare the mince and mashed potatoes as per the recipes elsewhere in this book.
4. Spread the mince evenly in the prepared baking dish, then top with the mashed potatoes.
5. Draw lines on the top of the mashed potatoes with the back of a fork.
6. Sprinkle lightly with parmesan.

Tip: this is also delicious with sweet potato mash mixed with white potatoes.

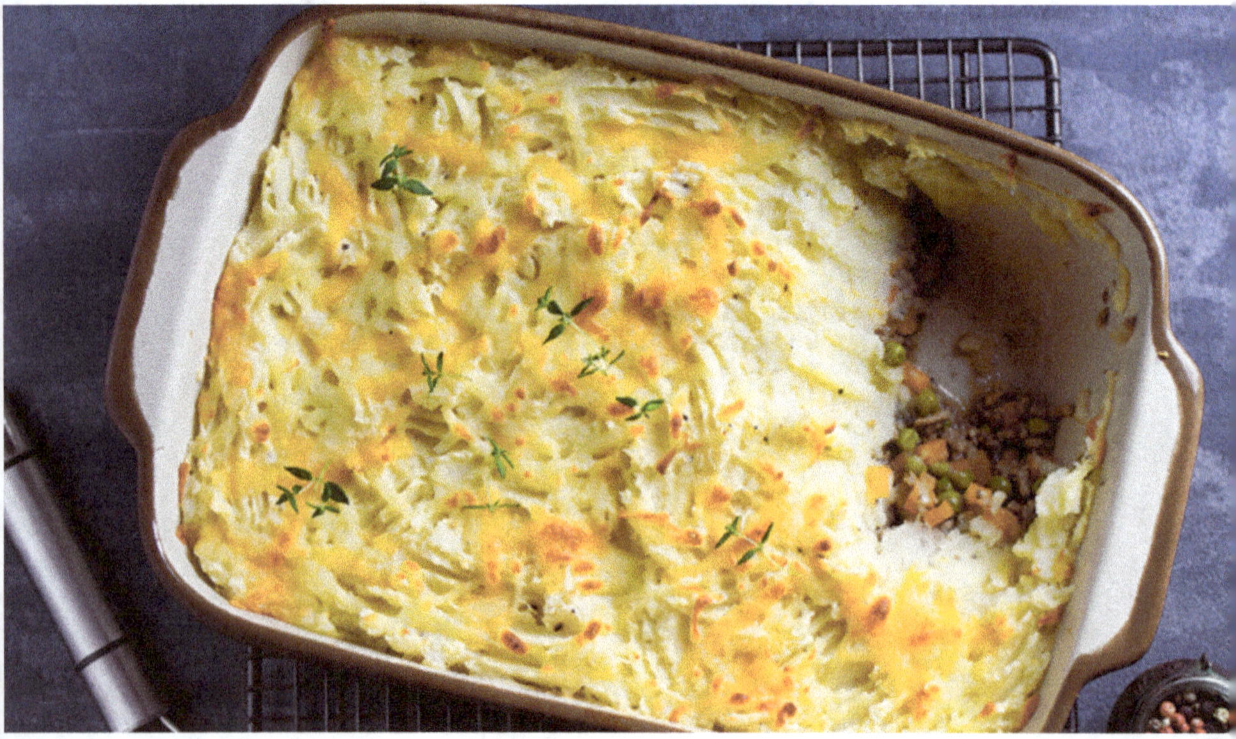

SOFT FOOD IDEAS *for* DINNER

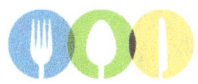

Pulled Pork – a Slow Cooker Favourite

Ingredients
- 1.5kg Pork shoulder
- 1 brown onion
- 2 tbsp brown sugar
- 1 tbsp ground cumin
- 1 tbsp smoked paprika
- 1 tsp garlic powder
- Salt and pepper
- 100ml chicken stock
- 100ml tangy BBQ sauce (store-bought)

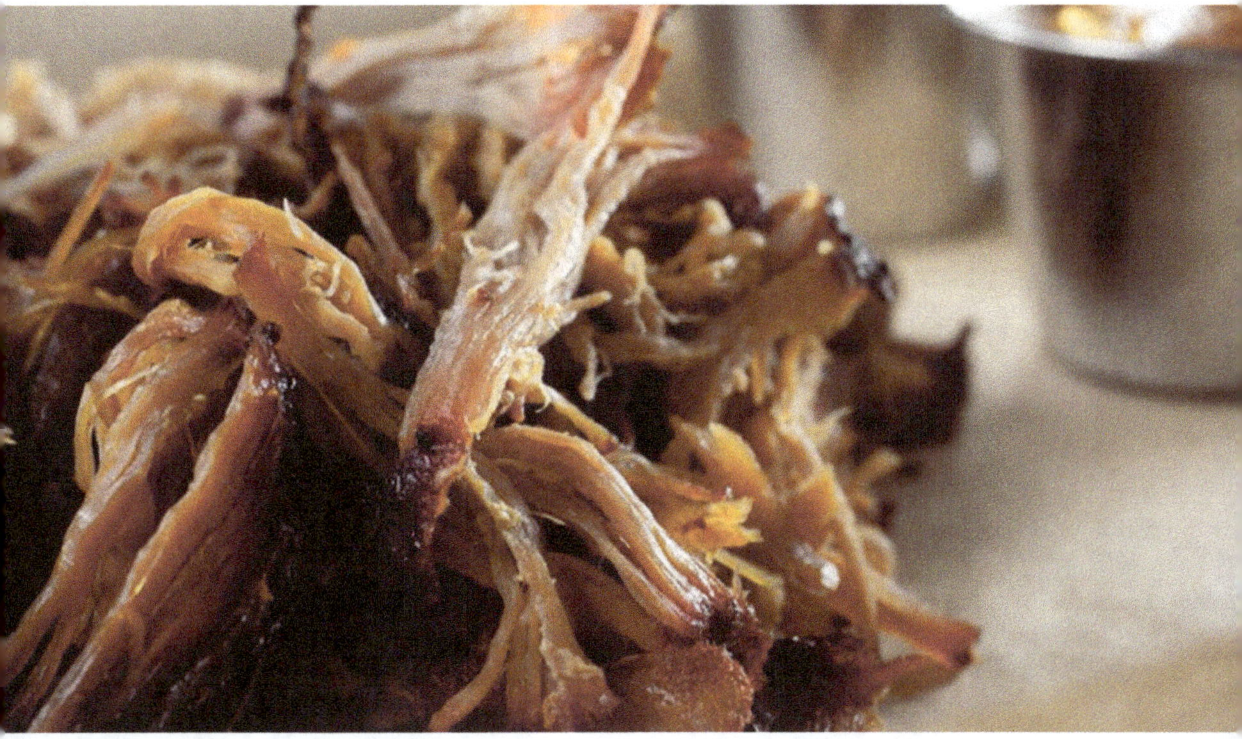

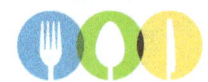

SOFT FOOD IDEAS for DINNER

Method
1. Slice onions and pan-fry lightly until cooked thru but only slightly browned. Remove and set aside.
2. Combine sugar, cumin, paprika, garlic powder and a good grinding of salt and pepper in a bowl.
3. Rub spice mix onto pork shoulder.
4. Pan-fry pork shoulder and brown all over.
5. Add onions to the slow cooker and place pork on top.
6. Add stock, then the BBQ sauce.
7. Put slow cooker on for six hours on low setting.
8. When ready, remove the pork and shred the tender pork using two forks.
9. Add the pork back into the slow cooker and toss with the onions and sauce. Add more BBQ sauce if required.
10. Serve with mashed potatoes and green peas.

SOFT FOOD IDEAS *for* DINNER

Roasted Sweet Potato, Feta and Basil Pasta Salad

Pasta salads are great for lunch, dinner and for packed lunches too!

Ingredients
- 500g Sweet Potato, peeled and chopped into 2cm cubes
- 250g pasta spirals (or any pasta you have on hand!)
- 100g Feta cheese
- 20g Basil leaves, shredded
- Olive oil, sea salt and cracked pepper

Avocado Dressing
- 1 ripe avocado, chopped
- 1 tbsp fresh lemon juice (optional)
- 2 tbsp extra virgin olive oil
- Salt and pepper

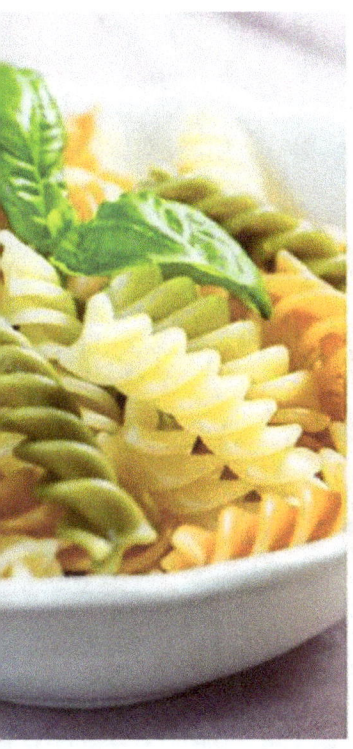
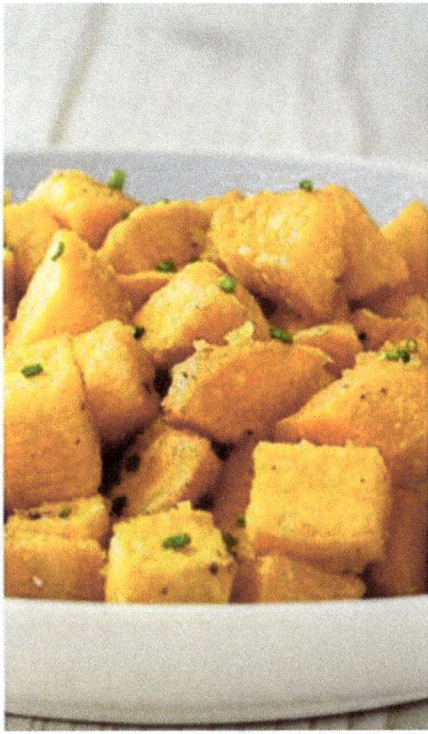
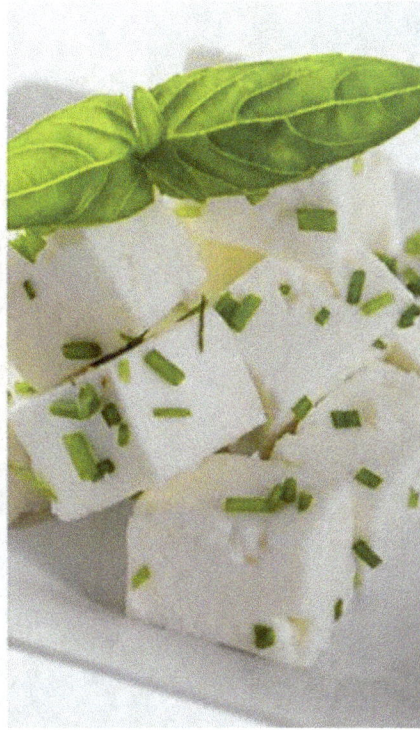

SOFT FOOD IDEAS for DINNER

Method
1. Preheat the oven to 200C & line a large baking tray with baking paper.
2. Scatter the chopped sweet potato on the tray, drizzle with oil, season with salt and pepper and toss with your hands until coated.
3. Roast for 20 minutes, or until lightly browned then remove from the oven and allow to cool.
4. Cook the pasta by following the packet directions.
5. Drain the pasta and rinse with cold water.
6. For the dressing, simply combine all ingredients in a blender or food processor and process until smooth.
7. Gently mix the pasta, roasted sweet potato and dressing until combined.
8. Sprinkle with crumbled feta and shredded basil.

Serving Suggestion:
Add cooked chopped chicken and kalamata olives for a Mediterranean feast.

SOFT FOOD IDEAS *for* DINNER

Bocconcini and fresh tomato pasta salad

Ingredients
- 300g Farfalle or Shell Pasta 220g Bocconcini (baby sized)
- 200g cherry tomatoes chopped in half or quarters 200g Spinach leaves
- ¼ red onion, finely sliced (optional)
- Honey Mustard Dressing
- 1 tbsp honey
- 1 tbsp extra virgin olive oil
- 1 tbsp white wine vinegar
- 1 tsp Dijon mustard
- Salt and pepper

Method
1. Cook the pasta according to packet directions. Drain and allow to cool.
2. Add bocconcini, tomatoes, spinach, onion and pasta to a large bowl and loosely toss to combine.
3. Add all dressing ingredients to a small bowl and whisk to combine. Season with salt and pepper.
4. Add dressing to pasta bowl and toss to combine.

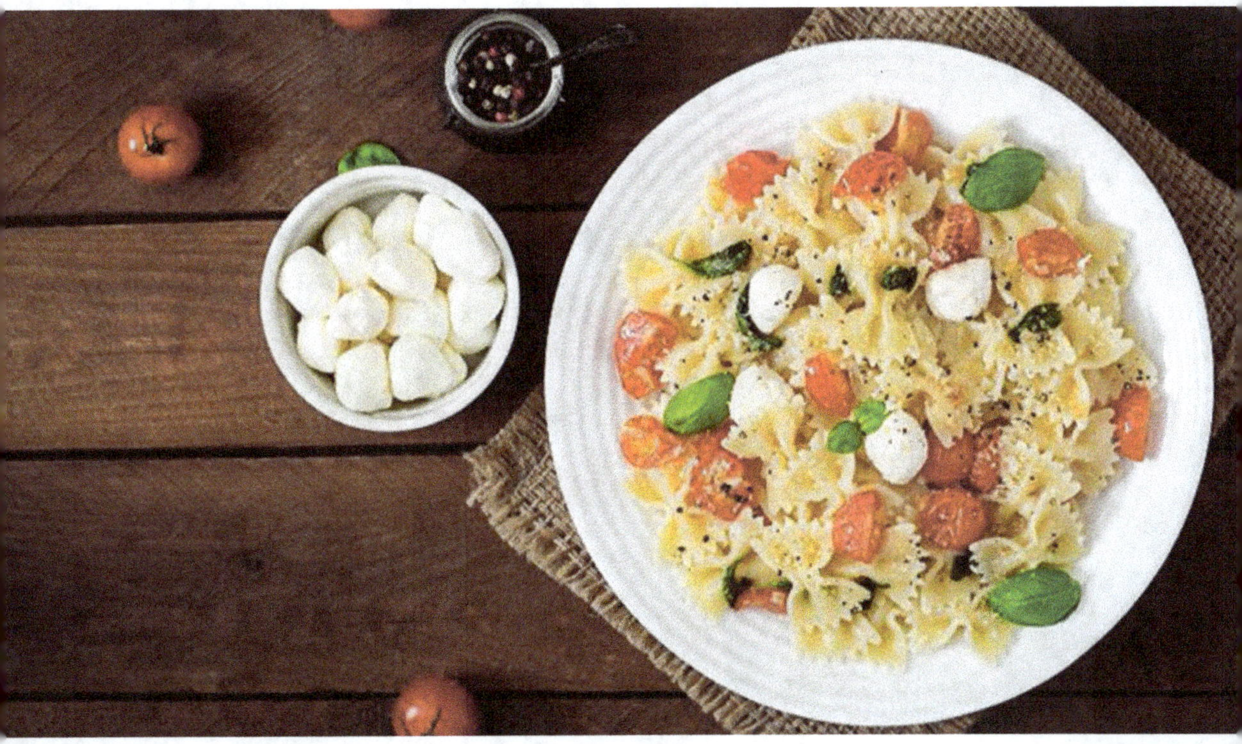

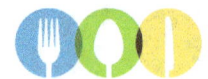 SOFT FOOD IDEAS *for* DINNER

DESSERT Recipes

Cottage cheese and chopped fruit – fast and easy

Ingredients
- 100g Cottage Cheese
- Small handful of strawberries or your chosen fruit
- Cinnamon
- Caster sugar (optional) or Splenda (sugar alternative)

Method
1. Spoon the ricotta into a bowl and top with chopped fruit.
2. Sprinkle with cinnamon and sugar and you are ready to eat!

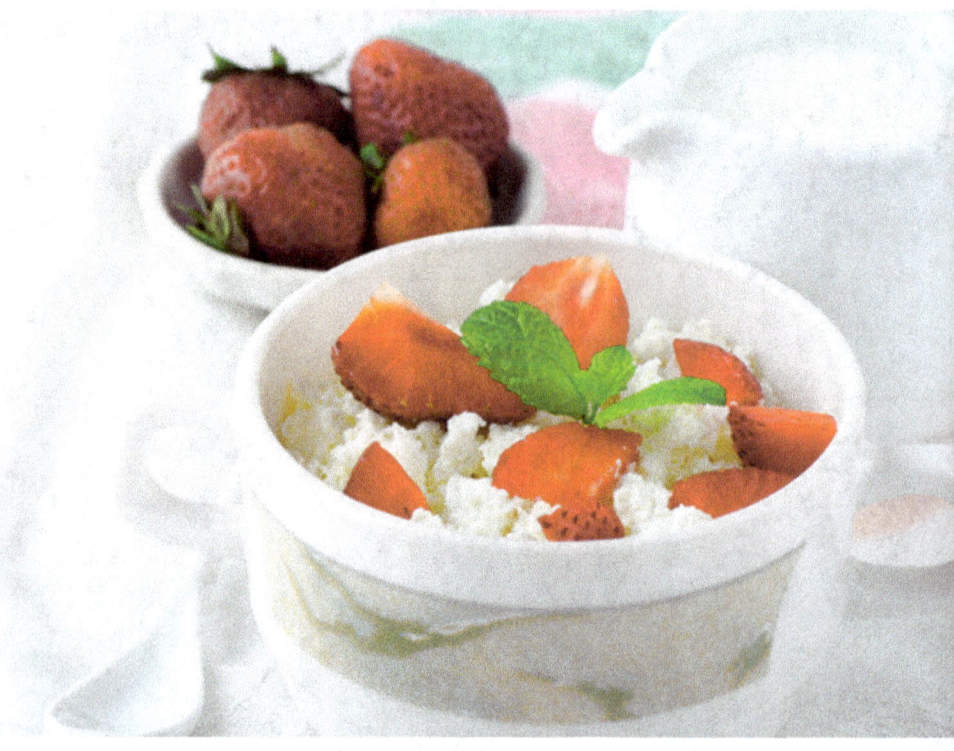

SOFT FOOD IDEAS *for* DINNER

Stewed Fruit – great for dessert or breakfast

Ingredients
- ½ cup water
- ½ cup caster sugar
- ½ tsp vanilla bean paste
- 1 cinnamon stick
- 250g strawberries or pears or apricots

Method
1. Add the water and sugar to a saucepan and heat until the sugar dissolves.
2. Add the vanilla and cinnamon stick, bring to the boil and simmer for 3 minutes.
3. Add your choice of fruit and cook on low heat for 3 to 5 minutes.
4. Remove the cinnamon stick.
5. Serve the fruit hot or cold.

Serving Ideas:
- Add a spoonful or two to the top of your breakfast porridge.
- Serve with ice cream, cream or custard for a delicious dessert.

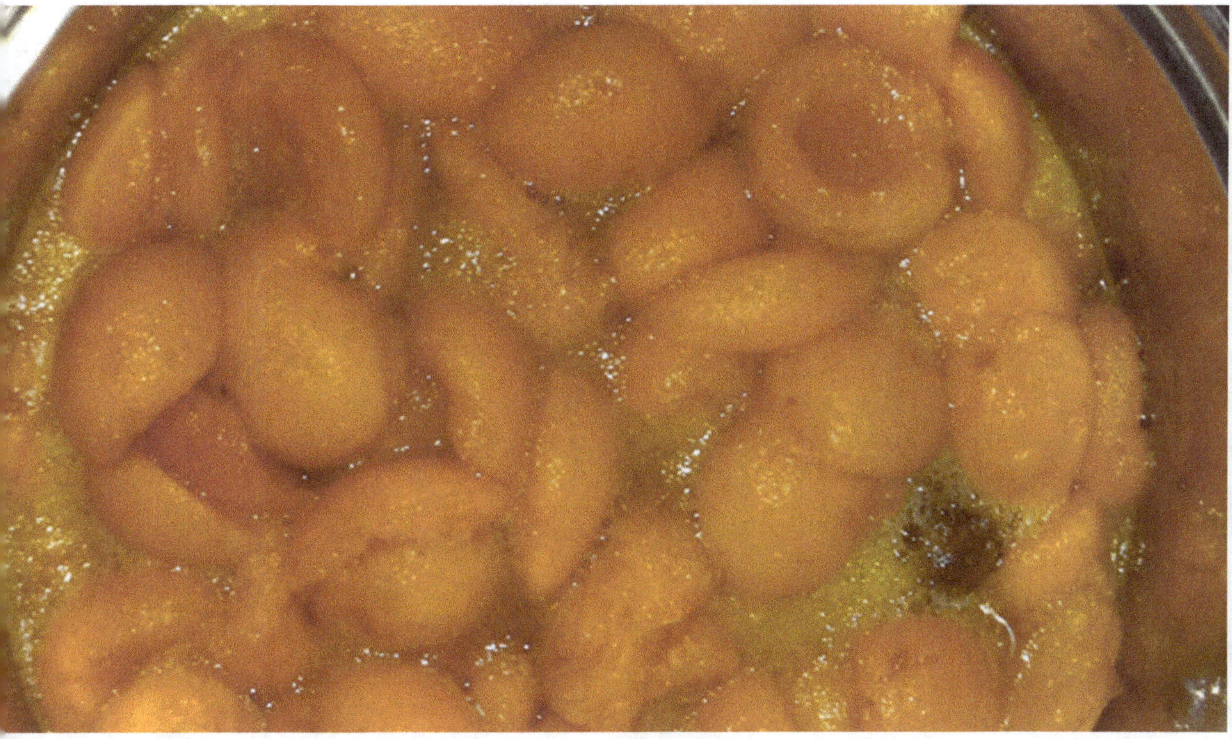

SOFT FOOD IDEAS *for* DINNER

Smooth Banana Dessert Bowl - a sweet delight

Ingredients
- 1 Banana
- 1/2 cup milk*
- 2 scoops vanilla ice-cream*
- 1 tbsp honey
- Drizzle of vanilla extract

Method
1. Put all the ingredients in a blender and whizz it up until smooth. So easy!

Tip: make this dairy free by using soy/almond/rice milk and replace the ice-cream with soy ice- cream.

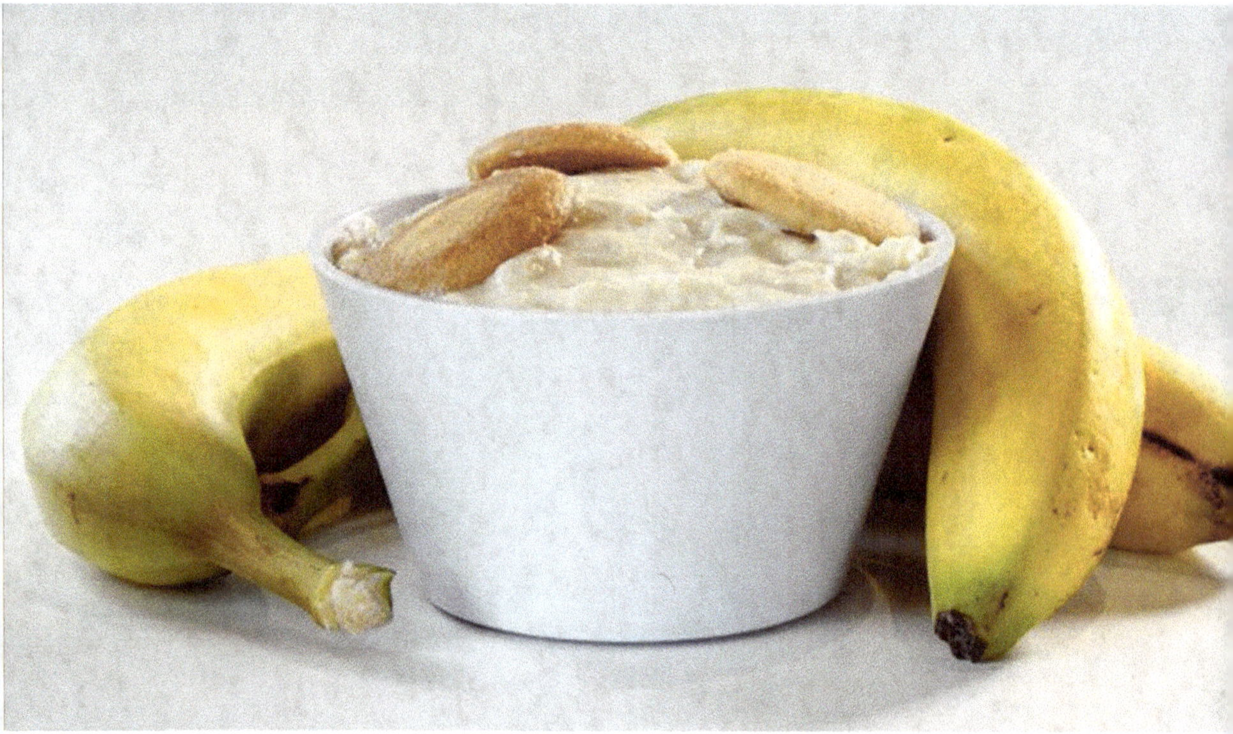

SOFT FOOD IDEAS *for* DINNER

Soft Cookies

These cookies are perfect to eat with ice cream for dessert, or pack and go as your perfect lunch box filler or snack on the run.

The secret to making cookies soft is adding milk and using mixed flours. Most cookies have the basic ingredients of flour, sugar and butter. The butter is effectively what makes them crunchy when baked. By adding milk (which is not usually found in cookies) and SR flour, we are softening the mixture and almost making a stiff cake mixture.

Ingredients
- 1 cup plain flour
- 1 cup SR flour
- ½ cup butter
- 1 egg
- 1/3 cup caster sugar
- 100g Choc Chips (optional)

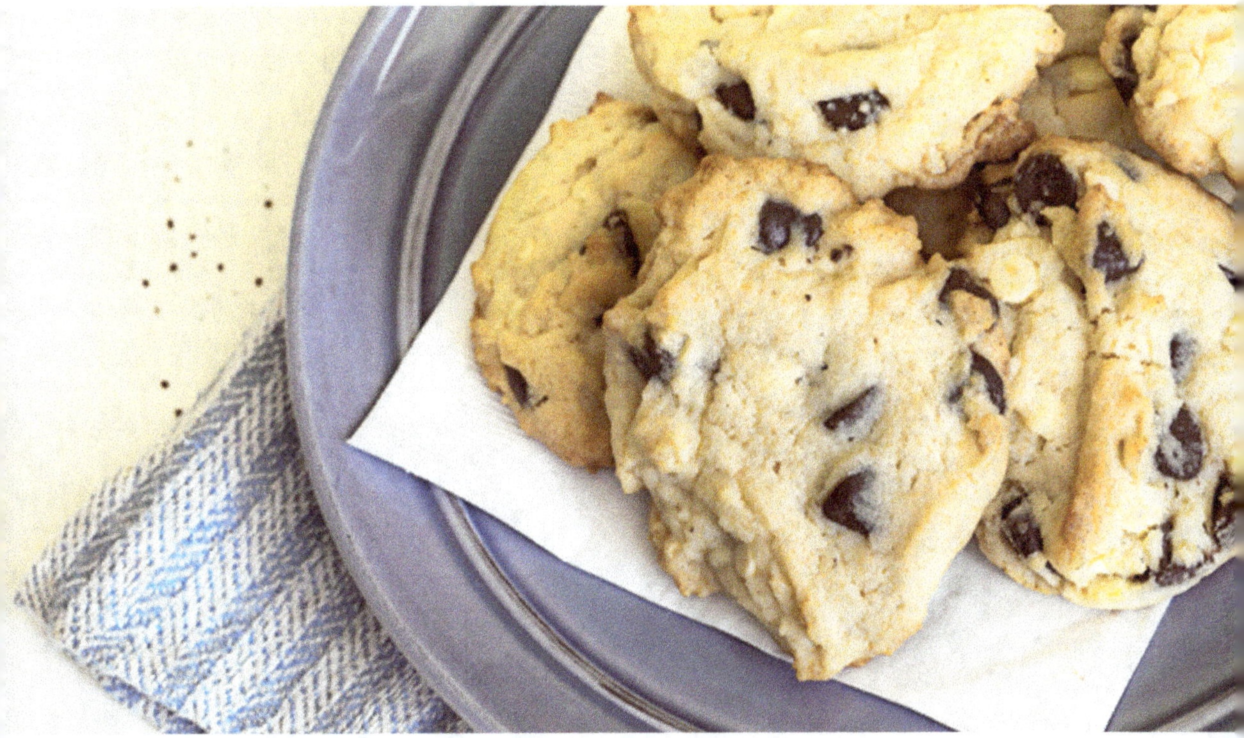

SOFT FOOD IDEAS for DINNER

Method
1. Preheat oven to 180 degrees Celsius and line a tray with baking paper.
2. Sift plain flour, SR flour and sugar together.
3. Microwave the butter until soft but not melted.
4. Whisk the milk, egg and butter together, then add to the dry ingredients and mix.
5. Add the choc chips (if using) and mix thru until evenly distributed.
6. Use a tablespoon to portion mixture, shape into a ball then flatten between your two palms until 1cm thick and place on baking tray, 2cm apart.
7. Bake for 14 minutes

SOFT FOOD IDEAS for DINNER

Apple Crumble - great for all the family to enjoy

Ingredients
- 6 to 8 Apples
- 1/3 cup raw sugar 1/3 cup water

Crumble
- ½ cup Self-Raising flour 80g butter
- ¼ cup raw sugar
- Sprinkle of cinnamon

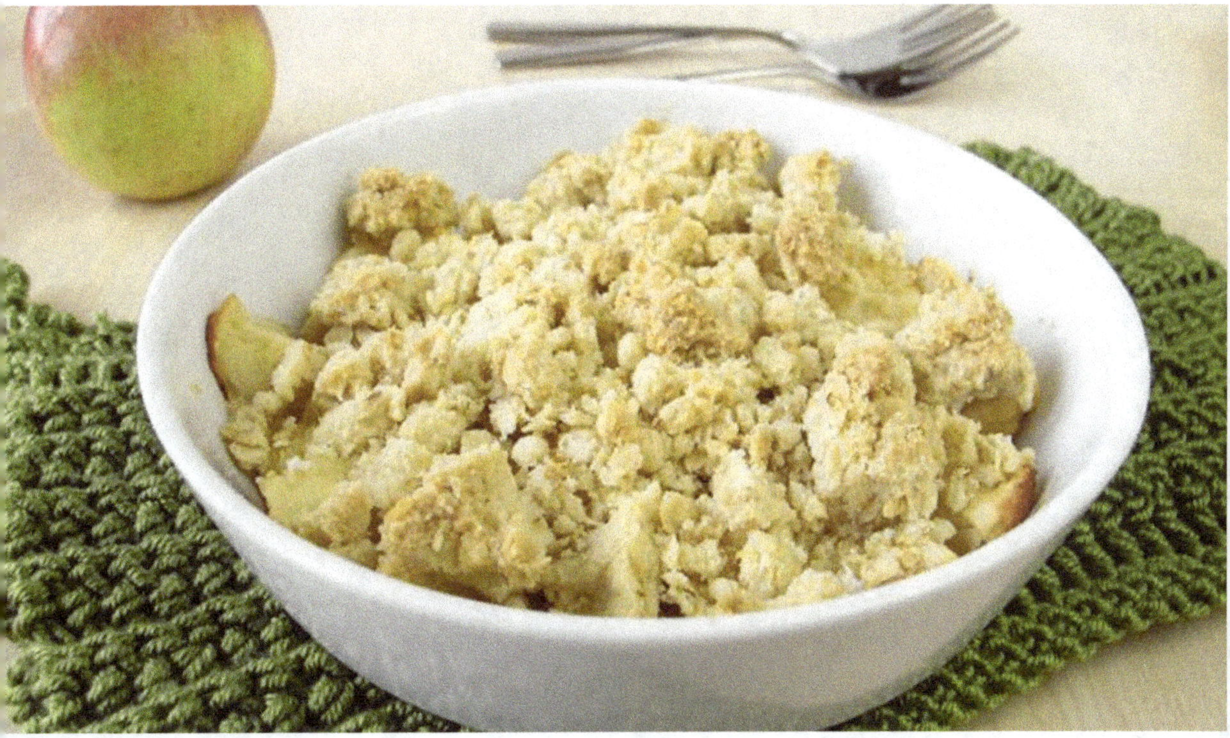

 SOFT FOOD IDEAS *for* DINNER

Method
1. Peel apples, slice off flesh leaving the core. Dice the apple chunks.
2. Add water, sugar and diced apples to a saucepan and bring to the boil, then simmer until apples are soft.
3. To make the crumble, melt the butter in the microwave.
4. Mix flour, butter and sugar in a bowl.
5. Tip apples into a baking dish.
6. Crumble the flour mix evenly over the top of the apples.
7. Sprinkle cinnamon over the top.
8. Bake in oven at 180C for 20 min or until brown on top.

Tip: This is a super easy recipe. Make sure you have a couple of peelers handy, put the music on and have fun making this one together with family and friends.

Serving Idea: Drizzle with runny custard and a scoop of vanilla ice-cream… yum!

SOFT FOOD IDEAS *for* DINNER

Self-Saucing Chocolate Pudding – chocolate heaven

Ingredients
- 2 cups SR Flour
- ½ cup caster sugar
- ¼ Cocoa
- ¼ cup melted butter
- 150ml milk
- 1 egg (optional)
- Canola oil for greasing

Sauce Ingredients
- ¾ cup firmly packed brown sugar
- 2 tbsp cocoa
- 1 ½ cups boiling water

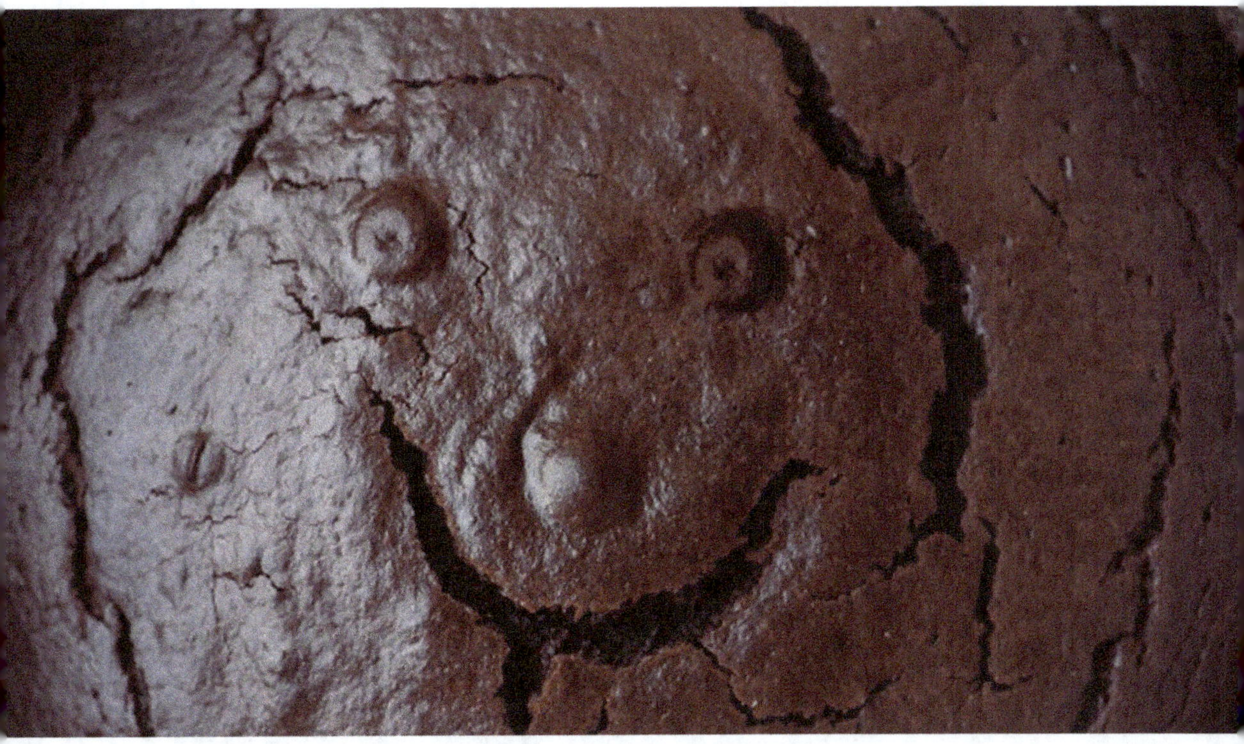

SOFT FOOD IDEAS for DINNER

Method
1. Preheat the oven to 180 degrees Celsius.
2. Grease an oven-proof casserole dish lightly with oil.
3. Combine dry ingredients in a bowl.
4. Combine milk and egg and whisk together with melted butter (after it has cooled or it will cook the egg).
5. Add wet ingredients to the dry ingredients and mix well.
6. Tip into the prepared dish.
7. To make the chocolate sauce, mix the cocoa and sugar in a bowl. Add the boiling water gradually, mixing to avoid lumps.
8. Gently pour the sauce over the batter.
9. Put in the oven to bake for 30 minutes. The cake will have risen to the top and the sauce will be at the bottom.
10. Serve hot with ice cream or cream. Simply delicious.

SOFT FOOD IDEAS *for* DINNER

Apple Pudding - You will be going back for seconds!

Ingredients
- 6 to 8 green apples
- 2 tbsp caster sugar
- 1/3 cup water

Cake topping
- ½ cup Self-Raising flour
- 1 cup milk
- 1 egg
- 2 level tbsp butter melted
- ¼ cup caster sugar
- ½ tsp vanilla extract

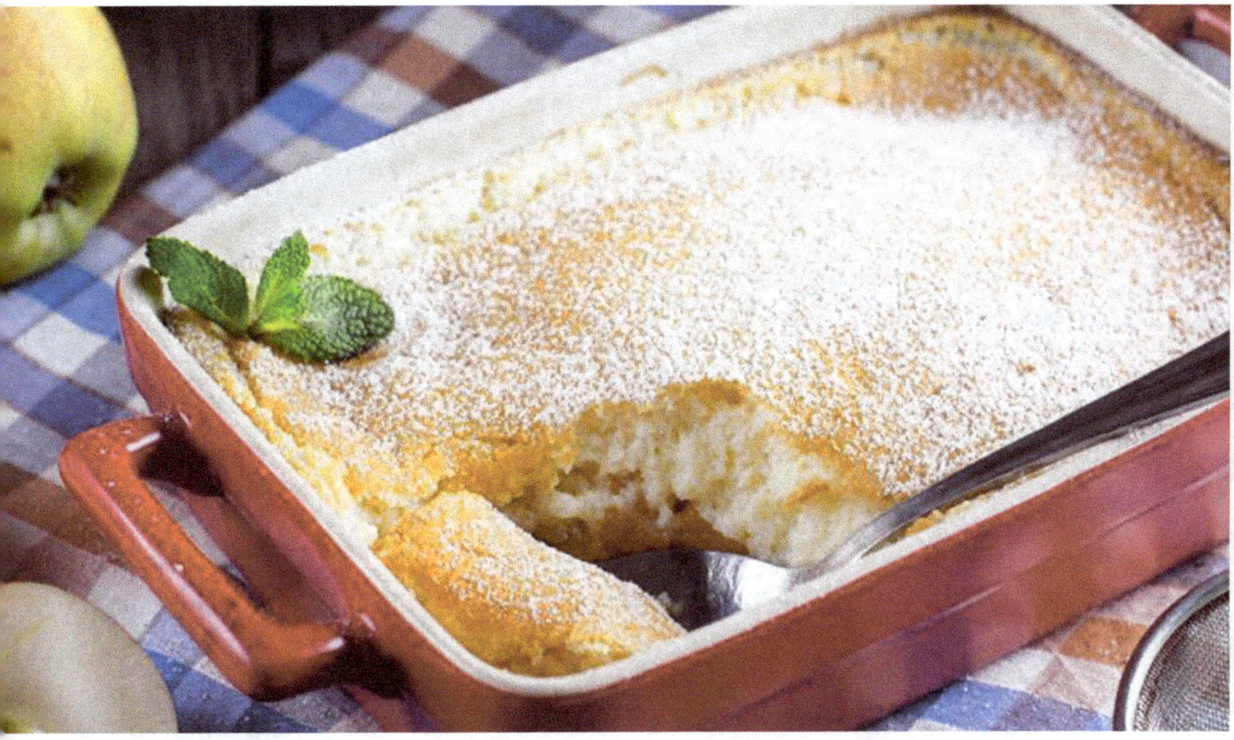

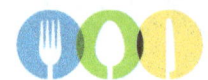

SOFT FOOD IDEAS for DINNER

Method
1. Peel apples and cut into slices.
2. Add water, sugar and apples to a saucepan, bring to the boil, then simmer until apples are soft.
3. Mix milk, egg, vanilla and sugar in a bowl.
4. Add the melted butter after it has cooled.
5. Sift in the lour and mix.
6. Place apples into a baking dish.
7. Pour over the cake batter.
8. Bake in oven at 180C for 20 min or until lightly browned on top.

Idea: substitute pears for the apples.

SOFT FOOD IDEAS *for* DINNER

Pear Clafoutis - sophisticated and delicious

Fruit
- 5 pears, peeled, cored and cut into quarters and halved again (into eights!)
- 1 tbsp caster sugar
- 1 vanilla bean pod
- 1 cup water

Batter Ingredients
- 1/3 cup SR flour
- 2 eggs
- ¼ cup sugar
- 1 cup milk
- ½ teaspoon vanilla extract
- Butter for greasing the baking dish
- 1 tbsp Icing sugar for dusting

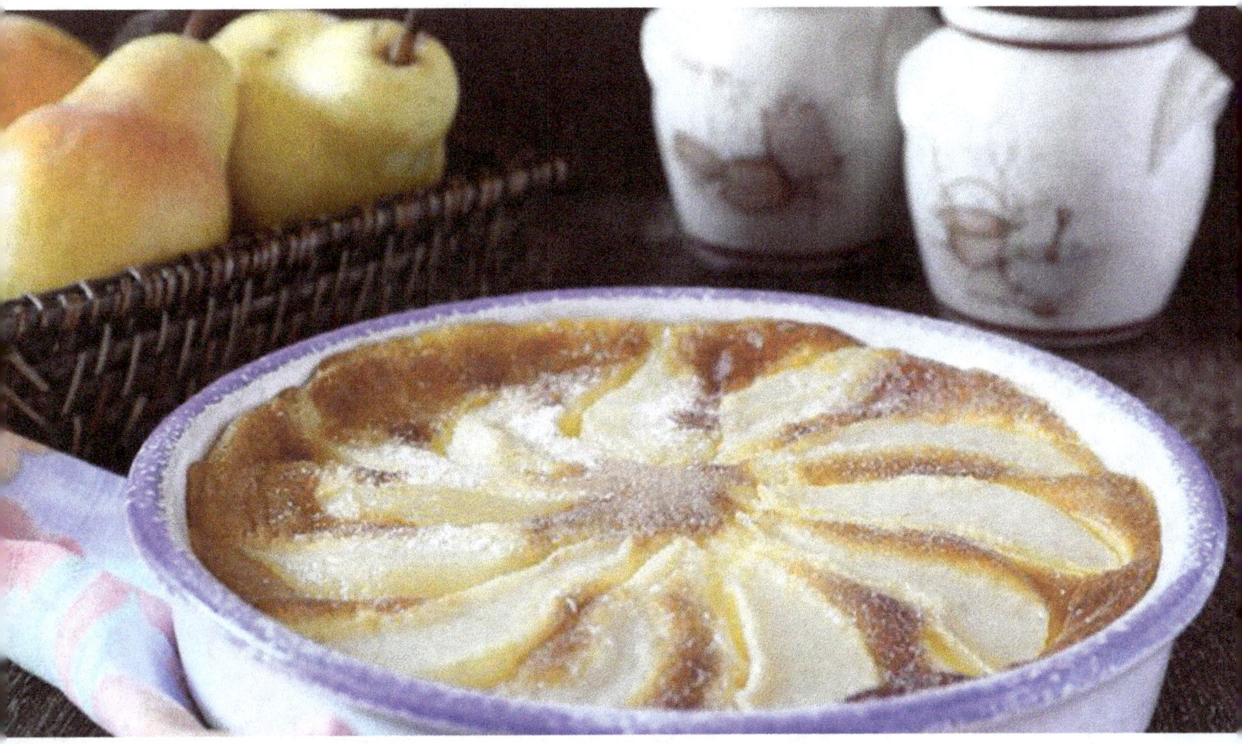

SOFT FOOD IDEAS for DINNER

Method
1. Preheat the oven to 180 degrees Celsius.
2. Scrape out a vanilla bean pod and add the paste to a pot with the water and pears. Cook until the pears are soft, turning occasionally and adding small amounts of hot water if needed. Once cooked, allow the pears to cool.
3. Mix the flour, sugar, eggs and milk together, then use a cake mixer to mix until smooth (no lumps!).
4. Grease a 20cm baking dish with melted butter.
5. Arrange the pears evenly in the dish.
6. Pour over the batter and place in the over to cook for 30 minutes or until a skewer comes out clean.
7. Dust the top with icing sugar and serve with cream or ice-cream.

SOFT FOOD IDEAS *for* DINNER

EASY Lunchbox Solutions

Packing a lunchbox to take to school, work or for travelling needs to consider temperature requirements. If you are taking dairy products or any food that needs to be kept at the correct temperature, you may need to pack an insulated container and/or cold packs. Some easy ideas:

- Chopped soft fruit – banana, melon, seedless grapes, kiwi fruit
- Cottage cheese mixed with diced strawberries and cinnamon
- Hummus (or other dip) with soft pita bread for dipping
- Yoghurt
- Pureed or diced fruit cups (store-bought or make your own)
- Muffins or cupcakes
- Slices of baked ricotta
- Thinly sliced lunch meats such as ham, polony/spam, turkey and potato salad
- Leftover pasta or pasta salad

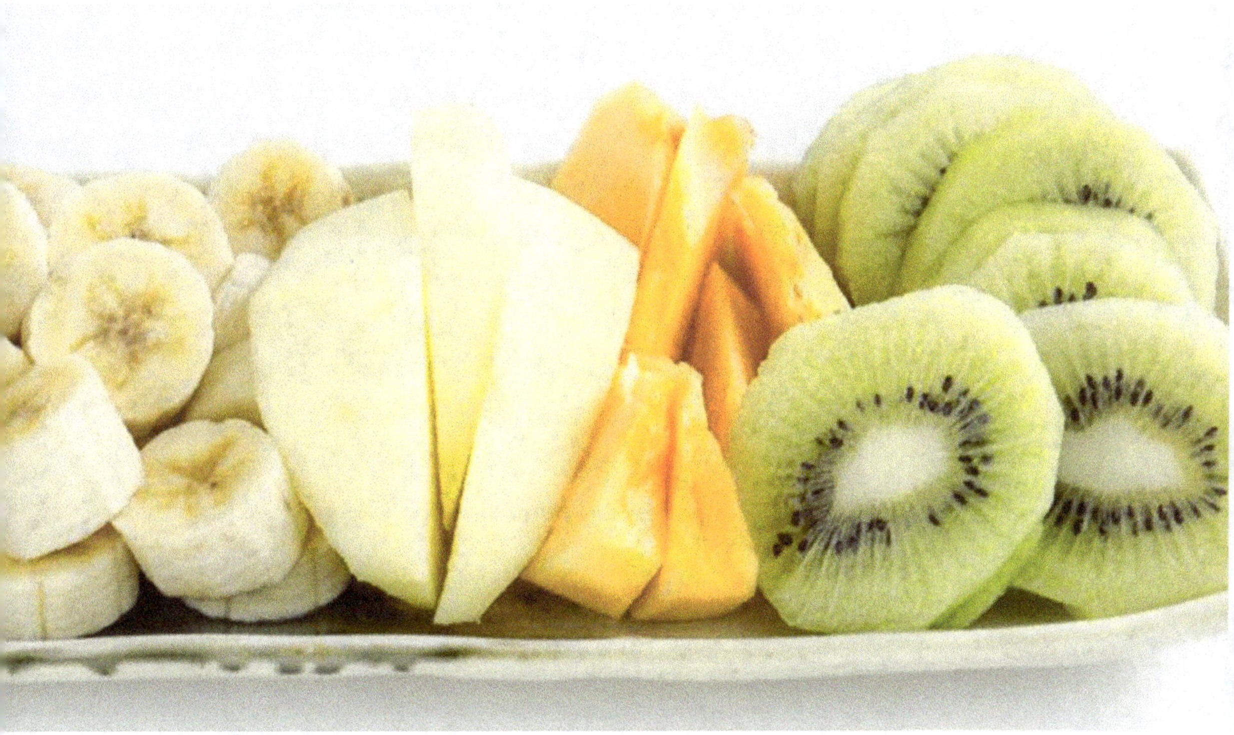

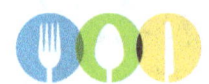

SOFT FOOD IDEAS *for* DINNER

Sandwiches

Use a soft style of bread and cut off the crusts. Go one step further and cut your sandwiches into smaller portions (triangles, tin soldiers or bite sized pieces) so your teeth don't have to work too hard.
Use fillings such as thinly sliced cold meats such as ham (avoid chewy meat such as prosciutto or salami), polony, turkey, leftover meatloaf, thinly sliced cheese or grated cheese and tomato, tuna and mayo, creamed cheese.

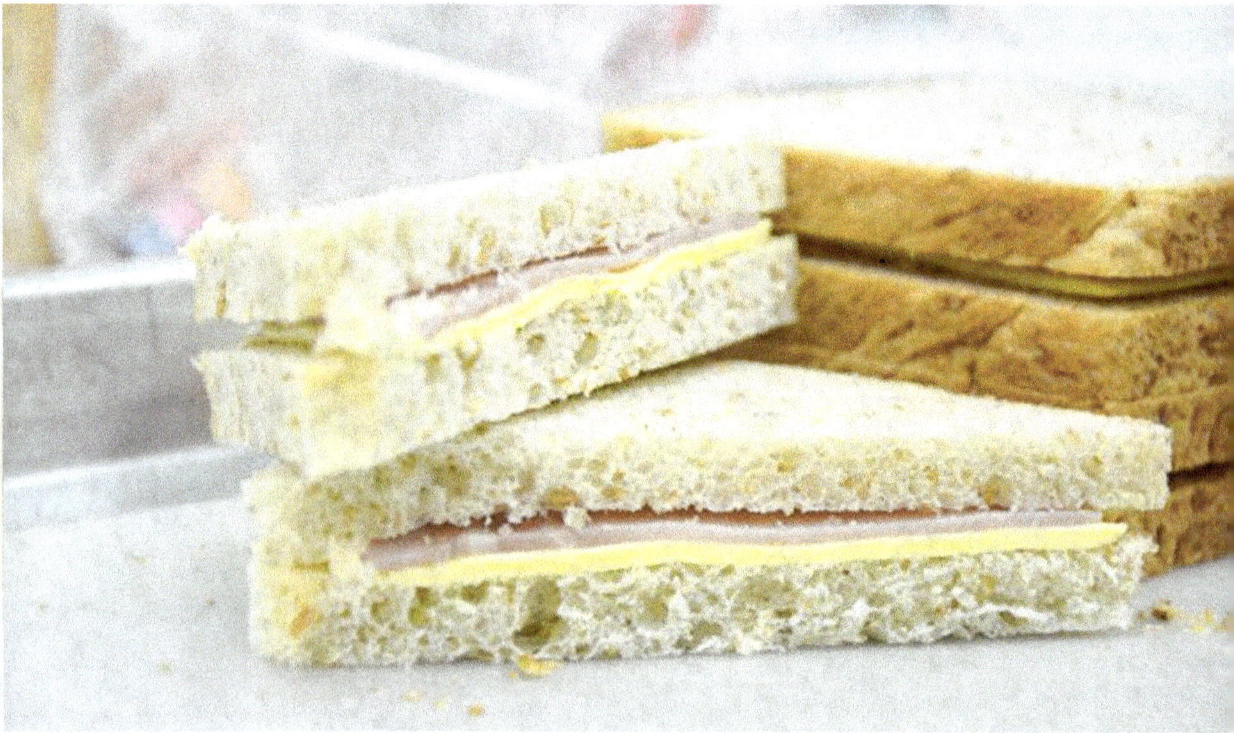

SOFT FOOD IDEAS *for* DINNER

Use your dinner leftovers

Lunch box ideas other than sandwiches are plentiful. In my opinion, the best lunch is always last night's leftovers! If you have access to a microwave, some of these options can be reheated for a hot lunch. Dinner leftovers could be any of the following:

- Soup
- Slow-cooked or stewed tender meat and vegetables
- Potato salad
- Pasta – if it was hot the night before, eat it cold and call it salad!
- Fried Rice or Risotto

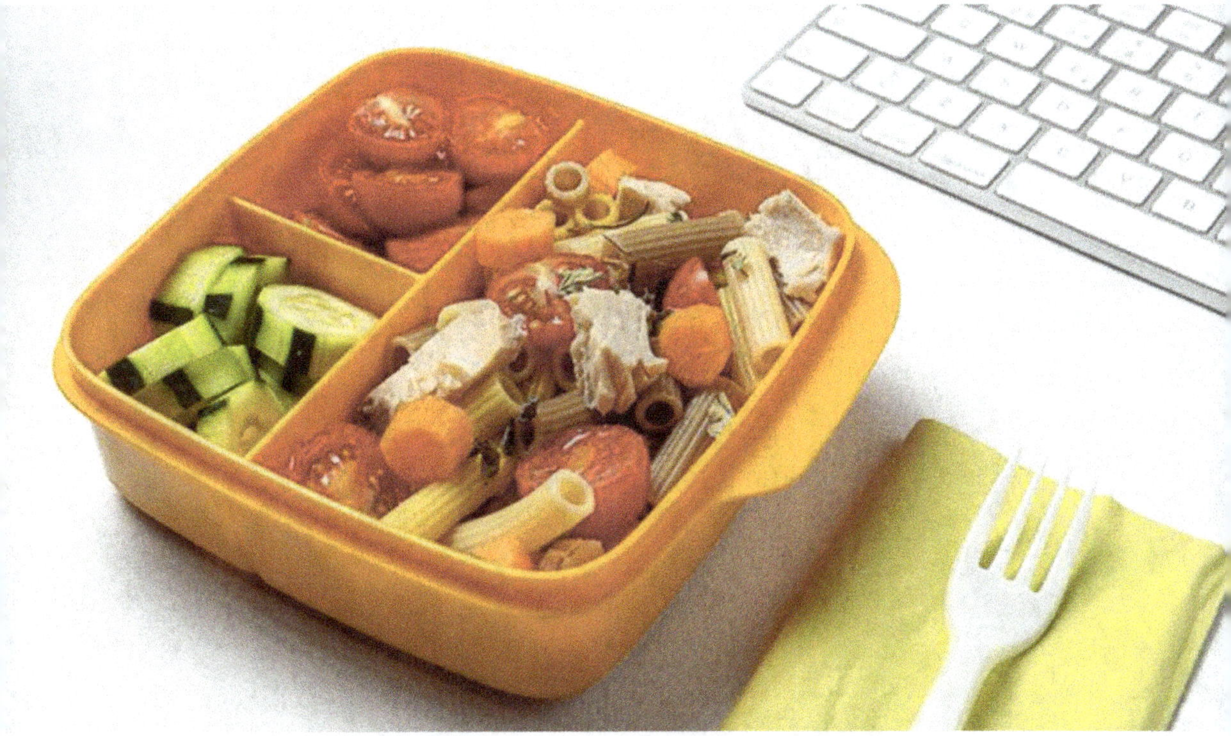

SOFT FOOD IDEAS *for* DINNER

Modifying Common Recipes for Soft Food Meals

Adapting your favourite recipes to suit a soft food diet can help make mealtime more enjoyable and ensure you still get to eat foods you love. Here are some tips and techniques for modifying common recipes to make them suitable for a soft food meal.

Pasta Dishes

Modification Tip: Cook pasta until it's very soft (a bit past al dente). Use smaller pasta shapes like macaroni or small shells.

Example Recipe Instructions: Creamy Macaroni and Cheese
Cook macaroni until soft, then mix with a creamy cheese sauce made from melted cheese, milk, and a touch of butter. You can also blend the sauce for an even smoother texture.

Casseroles and Bakes

Modification Tip: Ensure all vegetables and meats in casseroles are cooked until very tender. Cut ingredients into small, manageable pieces.

Example Recipe: Chicken and Vegetable Bake

Instructions: Pre-cook chicken until it's very tender, then shred. Cook vegetables like carrots, peas, and potatoes until soft. Combine with a creamy sauce and top with mashed potatoes instead of a crispy topping.

SOFT FOOD IDEAS *for* DINNER

Soups and Stews

Modification Tip: Blend or puree soups and stews to achieve a smooth consistency. Use soft vegetables and well-cooked meats.
Example Recipe: Blended Vegetable Soup
Instructions: Cook vegetables like potatoes, carrots, and squash until very tender. Blend with broth until smooth. Add cream for extra richness if desired.

Sandwiches and Wraps

Modification Tip: Use soft breads with the crusts removed. Choose fillings that are easy to chew, such as mashed avocado, soft cheeses, or egg salad.

Example Recipe: Soft Egg Salad Sandwich

Instructions: Prepare egg salad by mixing chopped boiled eggs with mayonnaise until creamy. Spread on soft bread with the crusts removed.

Breakfast Favorites

Modification Tip: Soften breakfast items like pancakes, waffles, and cereals by adding extra milk.

Example Recipe: Soft fluffy Pancakes
Instructions: Make pancakes with a batter that includes extra milk for a softer texture. Cook until lightly browned but still soft. Serve with fruit puree or yoghurt.

SOFT FOOD IDEAS for DINNER

Desserts

Modification Tip: Choose soft desserts like puddings, custards, and soft cakes. Avoid crunchy toppings or hard pieces.

Example Recipe: Soft Apple Crumble

Instructions: Cook apples until very tender. Top with a mixture of oats, butter, and brown sugar, but bake only until the topping is lightly browned and still soft.

Proteins

Modification Tip: Use cooking methods that tenderize meat, such as slow cooking, braising, or stewing.

Example Recipe: Tender Braised Beef

Instructions: Slow-cook beef with broth and vegetables until the meat is very tender and easy to shred. Serve with mashed potatoes or pureed vegetables.

SOFT FOOD IDEAS *for* DINNER

Tips for Eating Out AND Ordering Take-away

Going out for Breakfast or Brunch

Foods to Avoid:
- Breakfast burgers Bagels
- Toasted sandwiches
- Fried chicken (yes, some people eat this for brekkie!) Crusty toast or bread with hard crusts

Breakfast and Brunch are full of great options. Consider these great ideas:

- Scrambled Eggs
- Eggs Benedict
- Bacon is ok as long as it is not too crispy
- Pancakes and waffles
- Banana Bread
- Bircher Muesli (no nuts or dried fruit)
- Smashed avocado on toast (cut off the hard crusts before eating)
- Muffins (no nuts and avoid staining berries such as blueberries) Iced chocolate
- Coffee diluted with milk
- Fresh juices

SOFT FOOD IDEAS *for* DINNER

Japanese Food - tasty but can be sticky

Foods to Avoid:
    Sushi is yummy but the sticky rice can be a nuisance, Only eat sushi if you are able to thoroughly pick and clean your teeth immediately afterwards. Choose soft fillings such as avocado or omelette.

Foods to Avoid:
- Crispy deep-fried food
- Curry

Better Food Choices:
- Sashimi (raw fish - avoid squid)
- Teriyaki fish or chicken (chop into bite-size pieces) Miso soup
- Tamagyoki - Japanese omelette
- Udon noodles
- Ramen

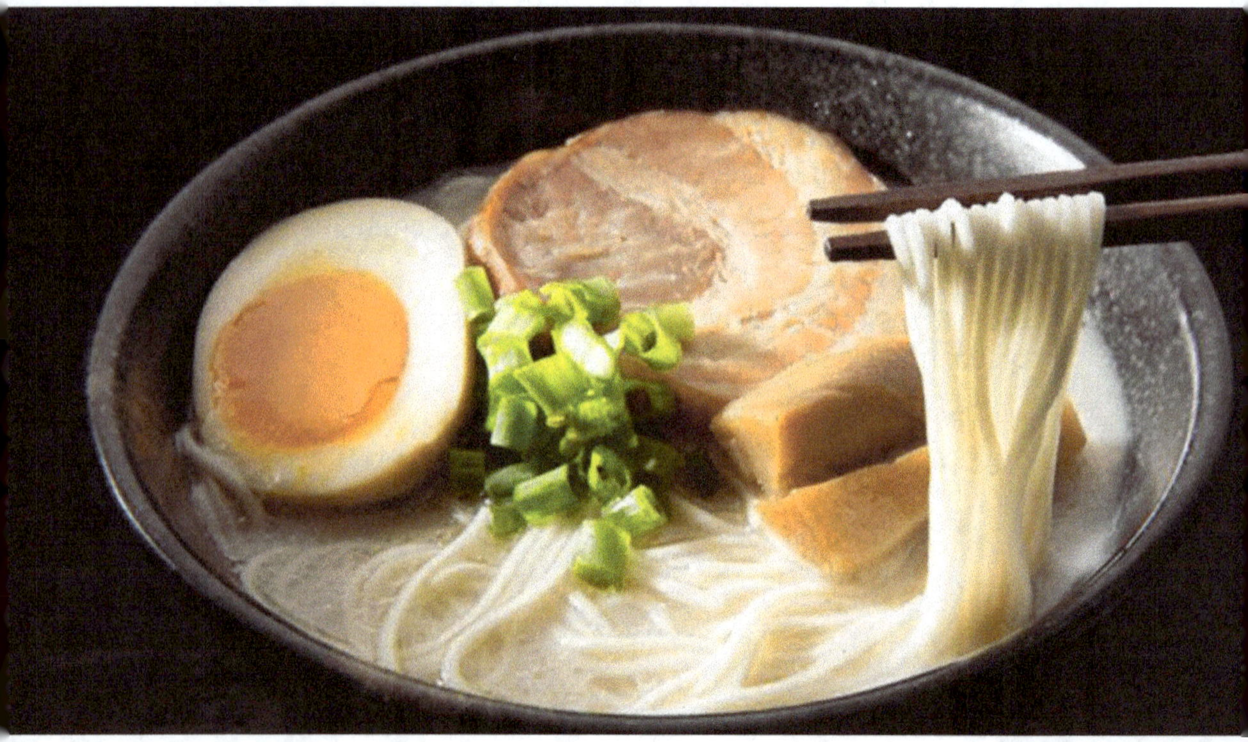

SOFT FOOD IDEAS *for* DINNER

Burger Joints

Burgers are big bite food. The action of taking a big bite of a burger can be difficult for a sore mouth and if you have braces, it will break them.

Burgers at home can be eaten using a knife and fork to cut the burger into small bite sized pieces. However, if you are out at a burger joint this might not be the best option.
Instead think about ordering potatoes wedges and avoid the crispy ones!

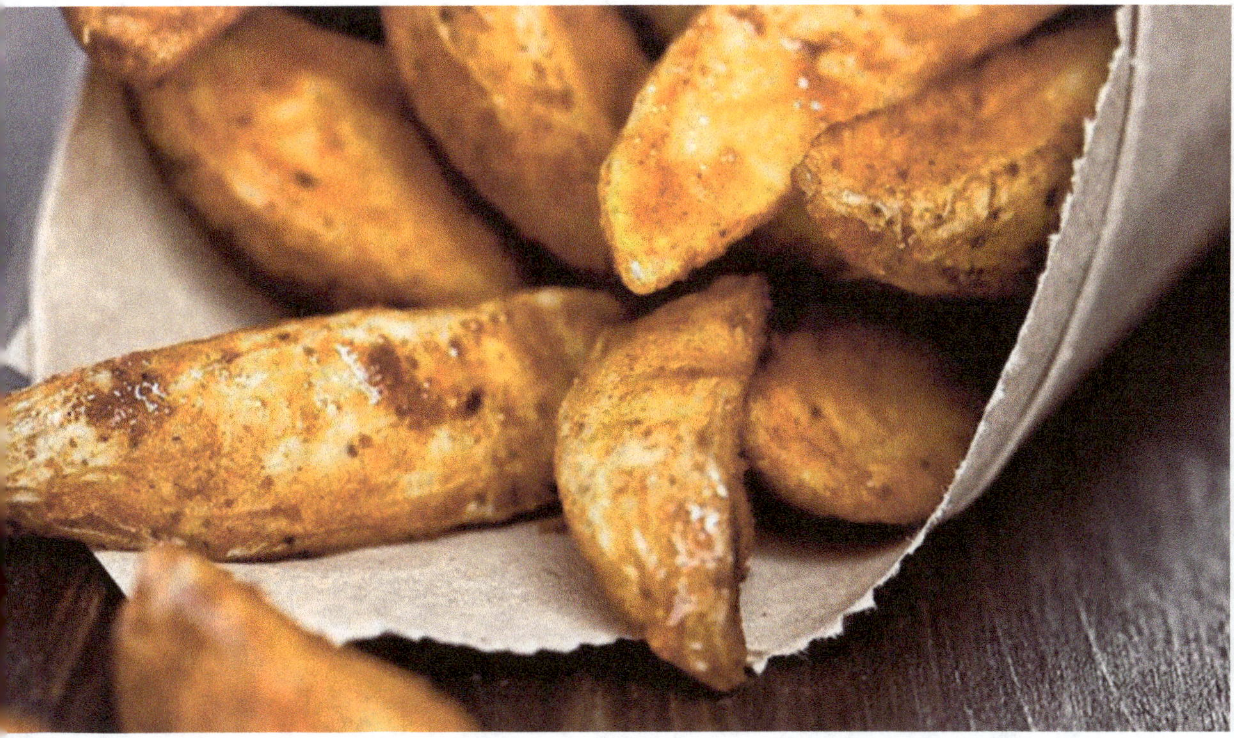

SOFT FOOD IDEAS for DINNER

Pizza - Eating out and Take-away

Avoid Hard Crusts on Pizza and instead cut the crust off the pizza and use a knife and fork to cut your pizza into bite size portions.

Also consider ordering a white-based pizzas that does not have the traditional tomato base, as the tomato base can cause staining.

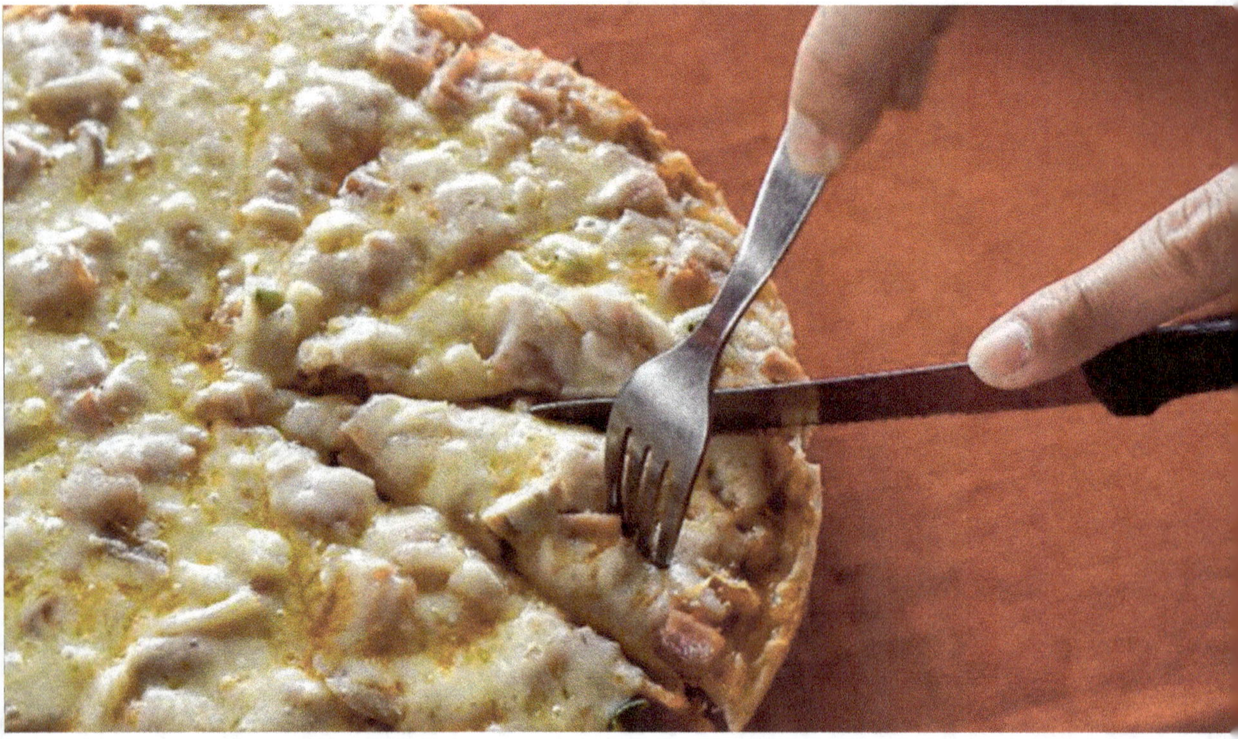

SOFT FOOD IDEAS *for* DINNER

Italian Food - creamy pastas are perfect

Avoid rich tomato-based pastas, these can stain your teeth, dentures and braces.

Go for creamy pasta options instead which are soft and easy to eat and will not stain.

Filled pasta such as ravioli or tortellini are also good options.
Garlic bread is fine, just chop off the crispy crusts.

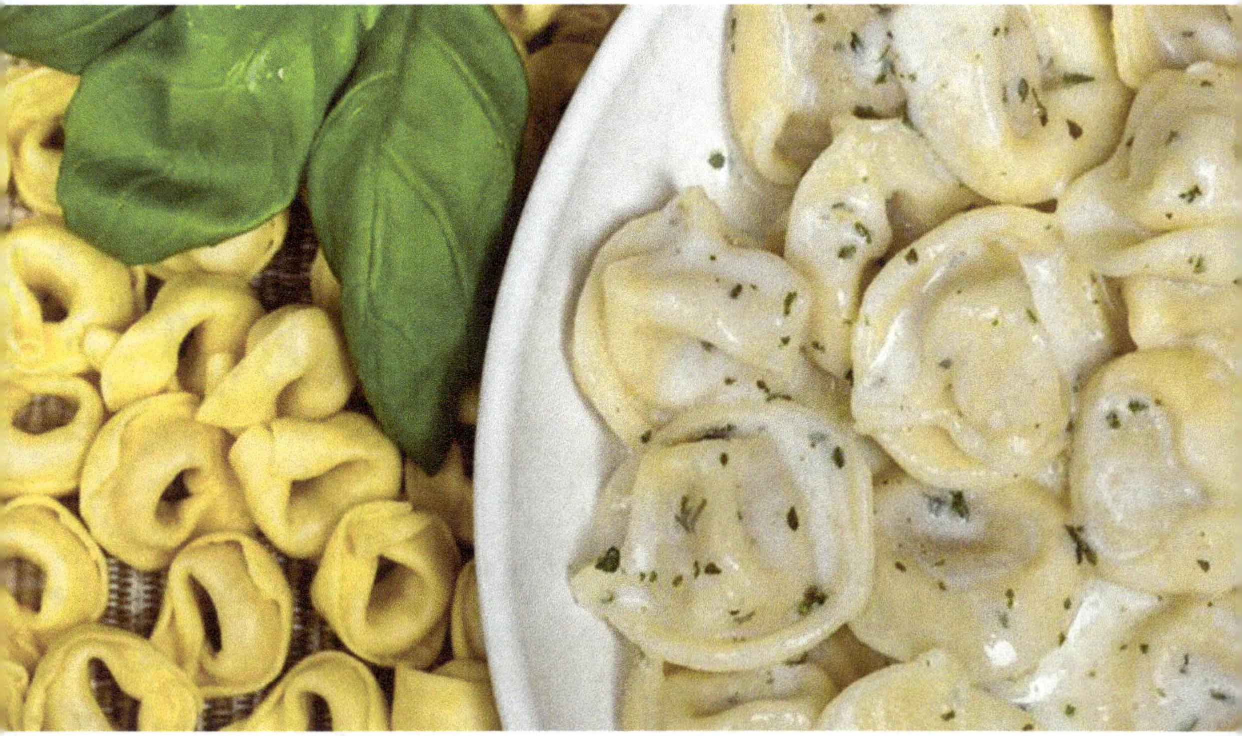

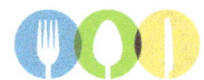

SOFT FOOD IDEAS *for* DINNER

Chinese Food - lots of great options

Some judgement is required with Chinese food due to the large and varied menu of food on offer. Avoid crispy fried food and nuts (sometimes included in stir-fry dishes).

Apart from that, Chinese food offers some great options as much of the food is already cut into bite-size pieces. Some easy options include:

- Chow Mein (with soft noodles not crispy)
- Omelette
- Fried Rice
- Steamed dumplings
- Scallops, prawns, chicken off the bone, fish (no bones)
- Stir-fry's
- Noodles

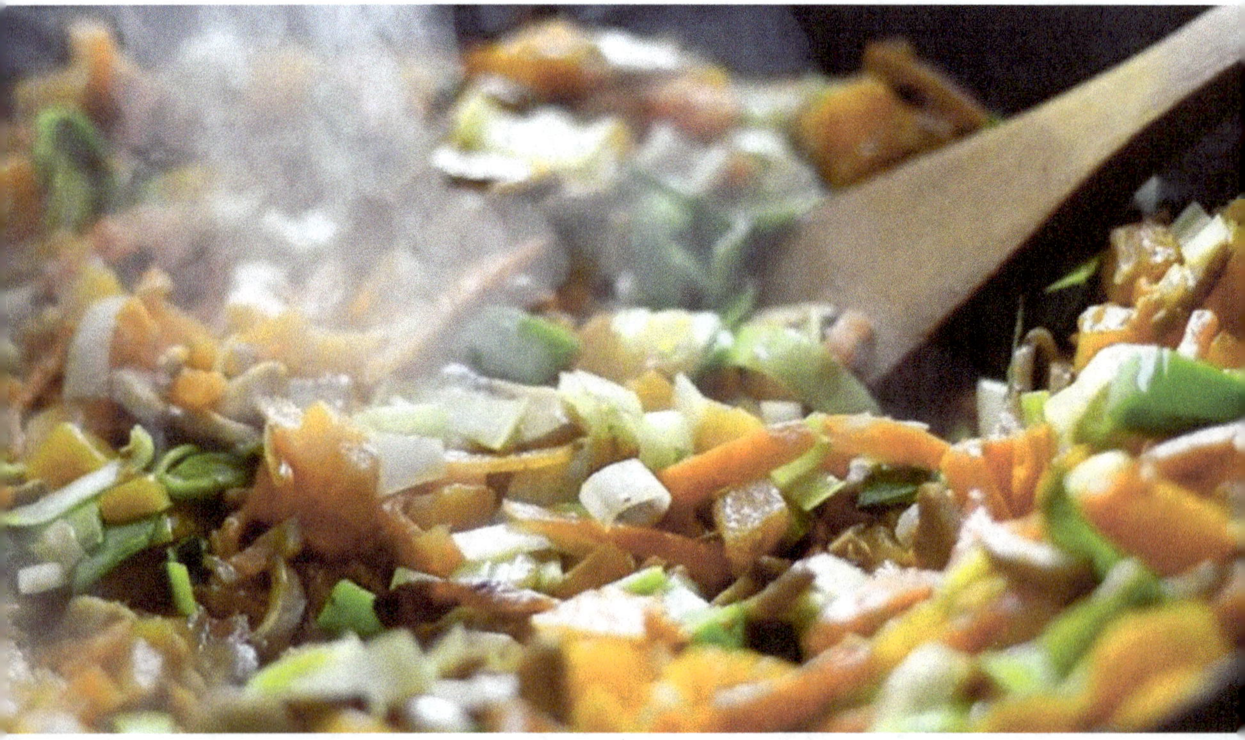

SOFT FOOD IDEAS *for* DINNER

Indian Food can be tricky

Most Indian food is rich in colour and flavour. Unfortunately, this is a problem due to potential staining issues. You will need avoid any dishes containing turmeric, rich tomato curries and tandoori.

A few safe (albeit limited) options include:

- Raita (yoghurt)
- Steamed rice
- Garlic prawns
- Onion bhaji (cut into bite-size pieces)
- Creamy cardamon based curries (no turmeric)
- Naan bread, chapati, paratha
- Mango lassi
- Gulab Jamun (sweet dumplings)

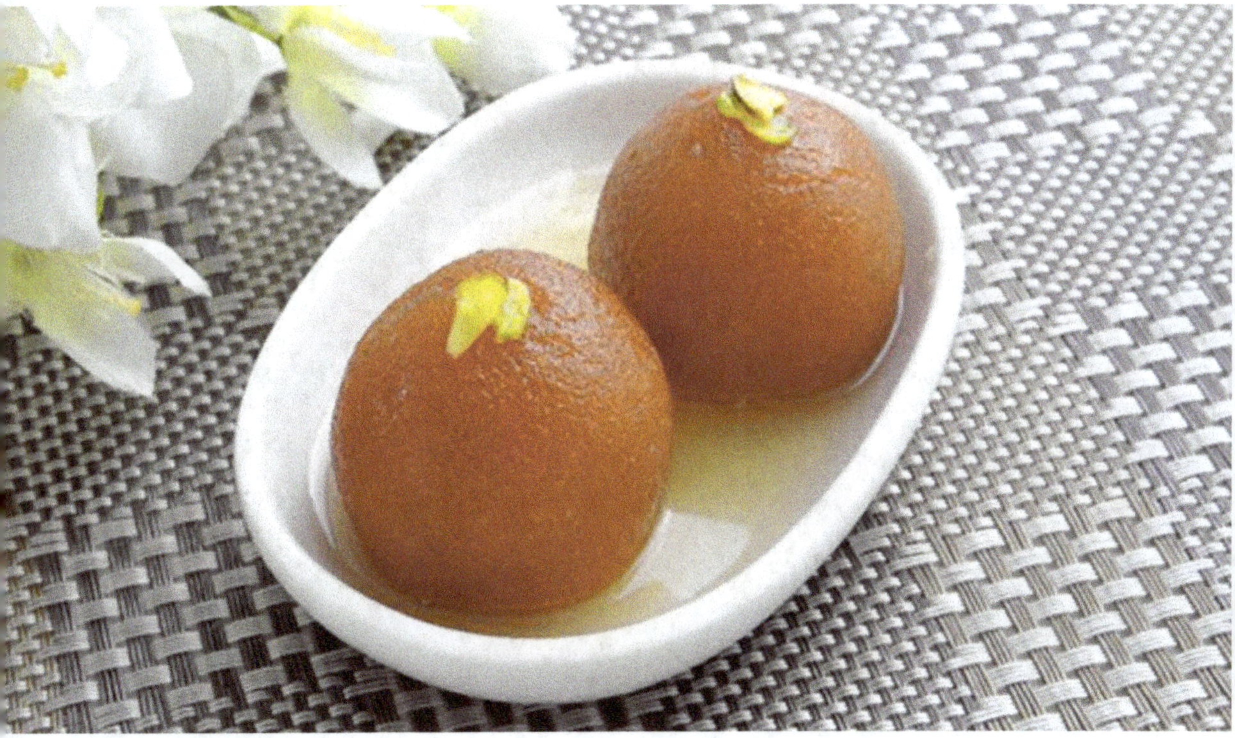

SOFT FOOD IDEAS *for* DINNER

Thai Food - some great tasty options

Avoid strong spices, crispy fried food, curries and satay dishes (which contains nuts). There are lots of great choices with Thai food! Consider these:

- Egg noodles, rice noodles, Pad Thai (noodles) – ask for your noodles without nuts.
- Stir-fries
- Pad Kra Pao Moo or Laab Moo - Minced pork
- Wonton Soup, Coconut soup, Tom Yum (spicy - avoid if you have sore gums)
- Fried Rice
- Omelette
- Steamed Fish and Fish Cakes

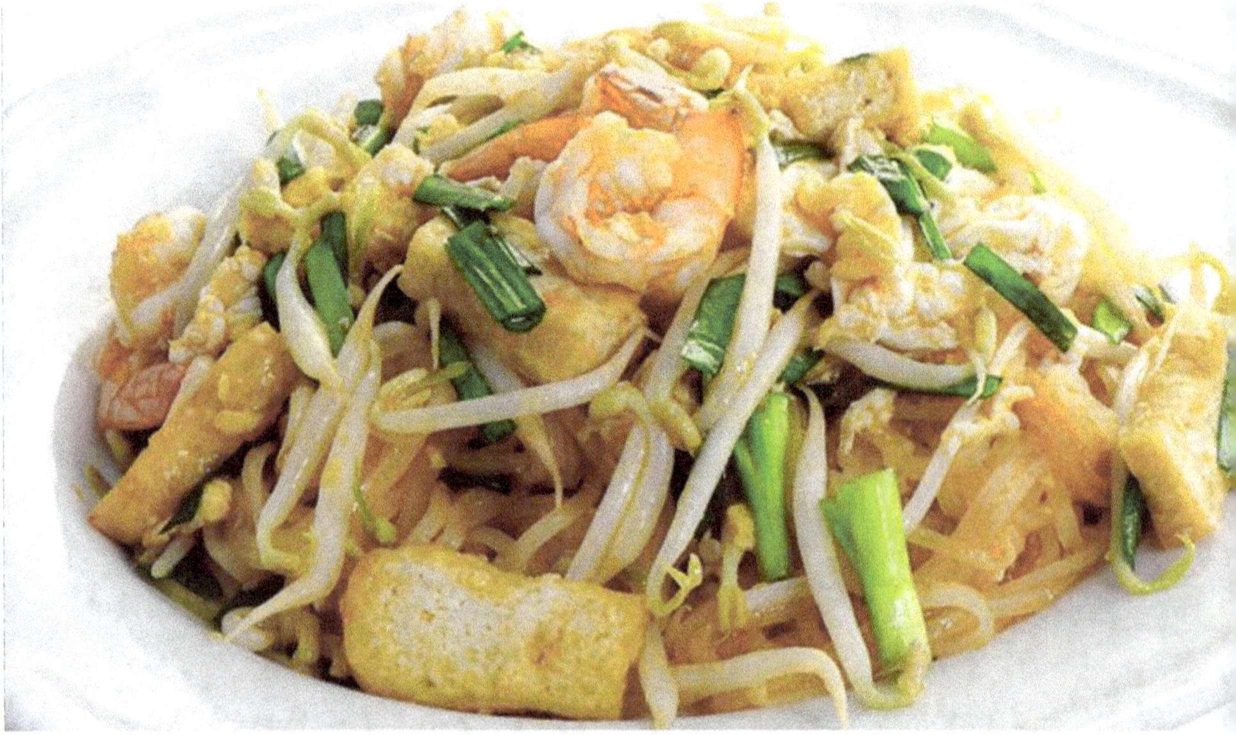

SOFT FOOD IDEAS *for* DINNER

American Food - avoid big bites!

Eating classic American food can be problematic as a lot of it is 'big bite' food which can be difficult to eat after a dental procedure or with a sore mouth. The following should be avoided:

- Ribs - avoid completely
- Hot Dogs
- Buffalo Wings
- Fried Chicken
- Reuben Sandwich

Better choices include:

- Burgers can be eaten with care. Do not take big bites. Cut into small pieces first.
- Meatloaf and spam
- Tub of mashed potato and gravy
- Chips/Fries - avoid hard, crisp ones Chicken nuggets
- Cornbread
- Macaroni and cheese
- New York Cheesecake

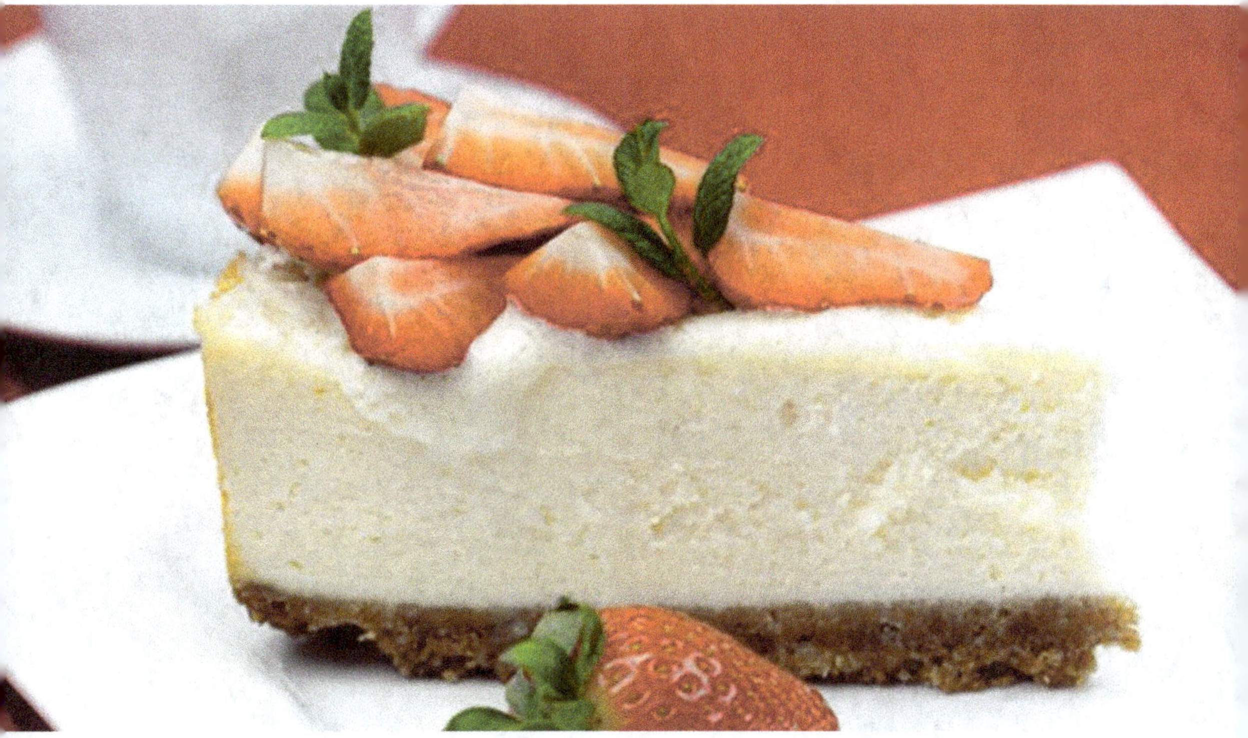

SOFT FOOD IDEAS *for* DINNER

Fast Food - What to Eat and What to Avoid

Food to avoid:

- Hot Dogs
- Burgers (unless you can eat with a knife and fork)
- Crispy tacos
- Kebabs
- Pizza Crust
- Fried Chicken

Better Choices:

- Chips – avoid crisp ones
- Burgers eaten by chopping into small bite-sized pieces
- Fish and Chips
- Chicken nuggets - cut or break into small bite-size pieces
- Tub of mashed potato and gravy
- Pizza - cut into pieces and avoid the crunchy crust

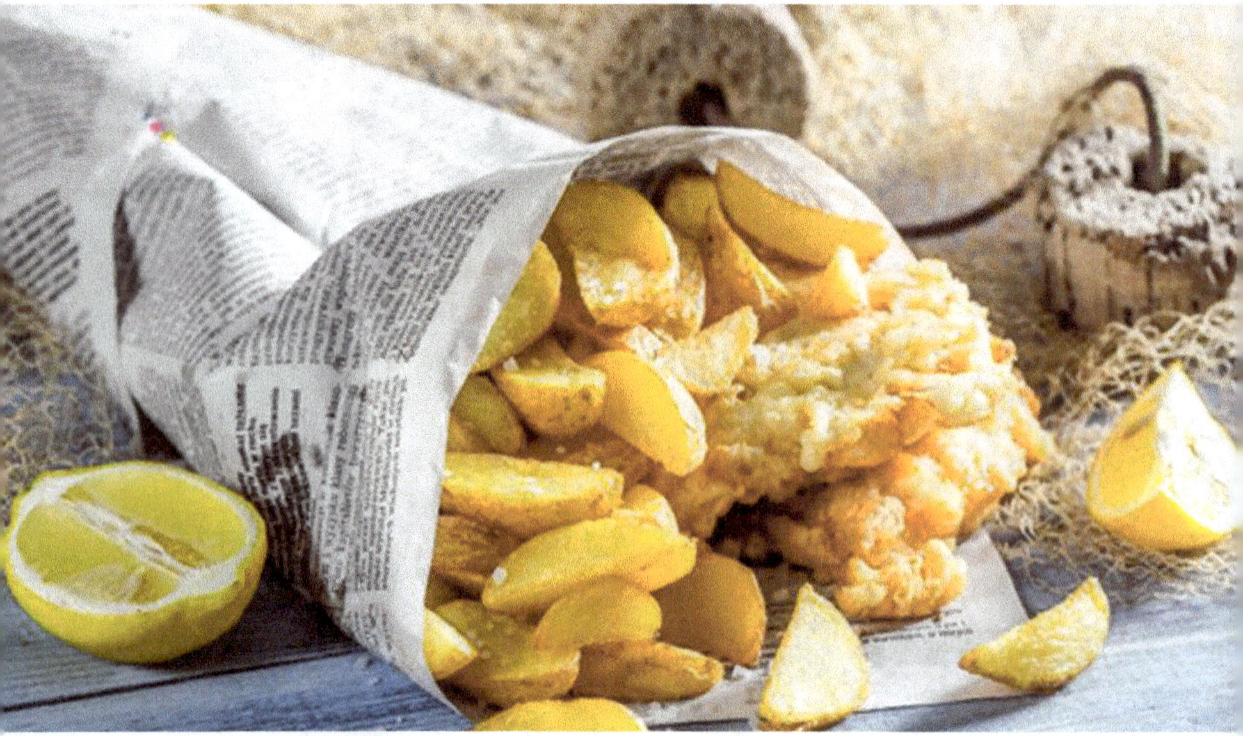

SOFT FOOD IDEAS *for* DINNER

Eating Out and Choosing Desserts

Avoid:

Avoid biting in churros and pretzels.

The good news is there are plenty of yummy options, such as:

- Ice cream and Gelato - avoid crispy cones and ask for yours in a cup Sundaes without nuts
- Trifle
- Donuts – break into small pieces Chocolate brownie (no nuts)
- Fruit salad - soft fruits (no raspberries or blueberries which can cause staining)

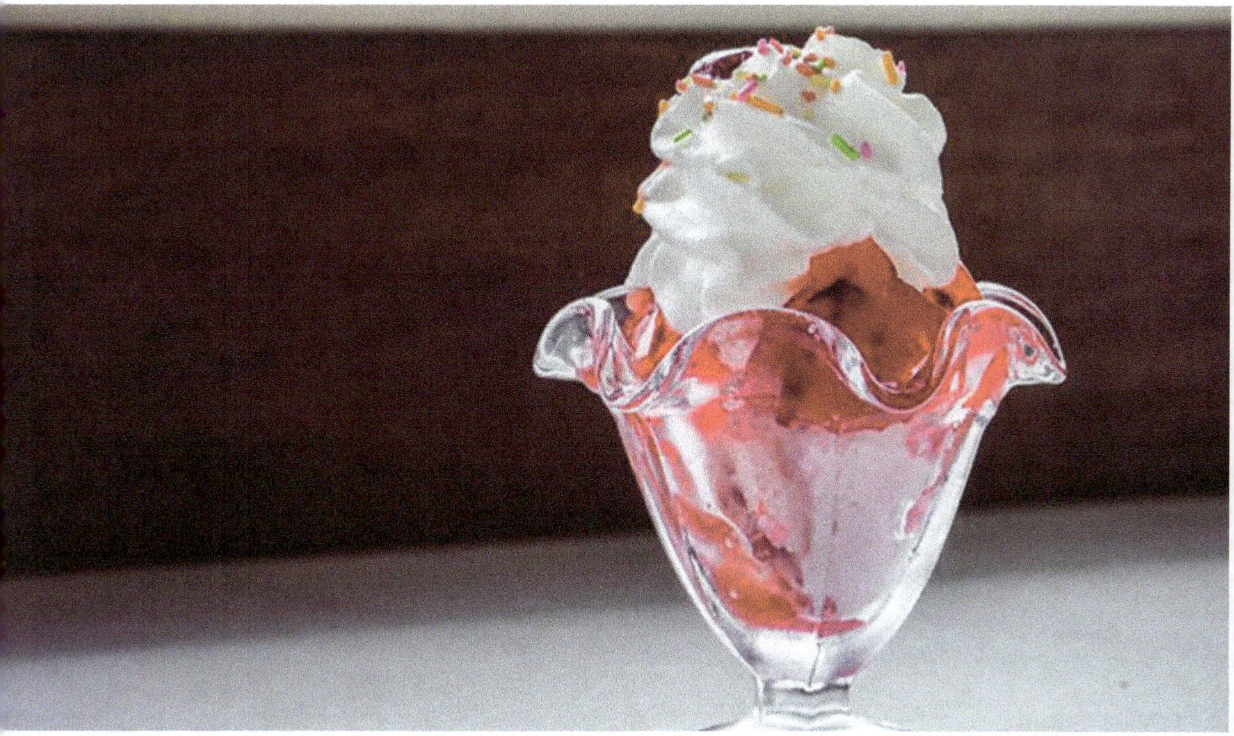

SOFT FOOD IDEAS for DINNER

Sample Meal Plan - First Week

MON	Breakfast – Banana Smoothie
	Lunch - Potato and Leek Soup
	Dinner - Mashed Potatoes and Gravy
	Dessert – Ice cream and jelly
	Snacks – yoghurt and apple sauce
TUE	Breakfast – Strawberry Smoothie
	Lunch - Potato and Leek Soup (double recipe)
	Dinner – Fish Chowder
	Dessert – Chocolate mousse (store-bought) and jelly
	Snacks – soft, chopped fruit such as banana, kiwi fruit
WED	Breakfast – Stewed fruit and Yoghurt
	Lunch - Potato and Leek Soup (made yesterday)
	Dinner – Roasted Soft vegies
	Dessert – Ice cream with mashed banana
	Snacks – Vanilla/chocolate cupcake
THU	Breakfast – Instant Porridge with stewed fruit
	Lunch – Chicken Noodle Soup (double recipe)
	Dinner – Salmon and Pea pasta
	Dessert – Crème caramel (store-bought)
	Snacks – yoghurt and soft fruit
FRI	Breakfast – Mango Smoothie
	Lunch – Leftover Salmon and pea pasta
	Dinner – Fish Patties and mashed potatoes
	Dessert – Ice cream
	Snacks – yoghurt and soft fruit
SAT	Breakfast – Banana and cinnamon mash
	Lunch – Chicken Noodle Soup
	Dinner – Savoury Mince and cauliflower cheese
	Dessert – Custard (store-bought) and soft fruit
	Snacks – yoghurt and apple sauce
SUN	Breakfast – Scrambled eggs
	Lunch – Leftover savoury mince
	Dinner – Sweet Potato, feta, basil pasta salad
	Dessert – Ice cream and soft fruit
	Snacks – yoghurt and apple sauce

SOFT FOOD IDEAS *for* DINNER

Sample Meal Plan – AFTER First Week

MON	Breakfast - Pancakes
	Lunch – leftover Sweet Potato pasta salad
	Dinner – Pulled pork and steamed soft vegetables with butter and pepper
	Dessert – Ice cream
	Snacks – fruit salad tub (store-bought)
TUE	Breakfast – Smoothie
	Lunch - Ham and cheese Sandwich (cut off crust)
	Dinner – Meatloaf, Mashed Potatoes and Gravy
	Dessert – Ice cream
	Snacks – muffin
WED	Breakfast – Pikelets with soft fruit
	Lunch – Sandwiches with leftover meatloaf filling
	Dinner – Baked salmon and cauliflower cheese
	Dessert – Chocolate mousse (store-bought) and strawberries
	Snacks – Pikelets
THU	Breakfast – Mushroom open sandwich
	Lunch – Salmon (leftover) and cheese sandwich
	Dinner – Pan-fried white fish with Potato salad
	Dessert – Apple pudding
	Snacks – Cottage cheese and chopped fruit
FRI	Breakfast – Smoothie of your choice
	Lunch - Potato salad and sliced turkey ribbons
	Dinner – Takeout night! Your choice of a creamy Italian pasta or a tasty Japanese ramen
	Dessert – Apple pudding leftover from last night
	Snacks – soft pita bread with hummus dip (store-bought)
SAT	Breakfast – Scrambled eggs with salmon
	Lunch – Macaroni cheese
	Dinner – Cottage pie
	Dessert – Apple or Pear crumble
	Snacks – muffin
SUN	Breakfast – Instant Porridge with stewed fruit
	Lunch – Sandwich with chopped boiled egg
	Dinner – Chicken and Noodle stir fry
	Dessert – Chocolate pudding and cream
	Snacks – soft cookies

 SOFT FOOD IDEAS *for* DINNER

About the Author

Suzanne Burke is a seasoned business professional with over 30 years of diverse experience across multiple industries, including mining, construction, government, media, banking, and information services, both in Australia and internationally. Her career began as a Computer Programmer and she diversified into roles such as Business Systems Analyst, Technical Writer, Small Business Manager, Digital Creator and Author.

With degrees in Information Technology and Professional Writing, Suzanne possesses a unique ability to cut through noise and clutter to assess any business or situation with clarity and purpose. She is adept at understanding the **"THE WHY"** behind issues and implementing **"THE HOW"** to find the most efficient and practical solutions. This combination of analytical and technical skills has earned her multiple business awards, showcasing her exceptional business acumen.

As an author, Suzanne has written two successful books: ***"Nail Your Renovation without Getting Screwed"*** and ***"Food for Braces."*** Her writing has been featured in publications such as The West Australian Newspaper, Money Magazine, Your Investment Property, Home Design, Better Homes and Gardens, New Idea and Woman's Day.

Suzanne's ability to create engaging, informative content that resonates with her audience has made her a respected author and a sought-after expert within the digital marketplace.

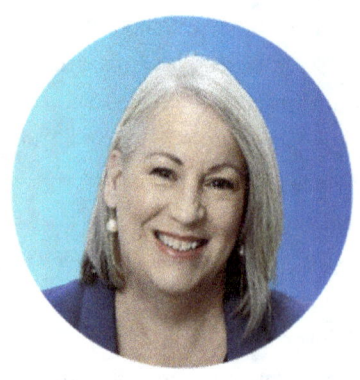

www.ingramcontent.com/pod-product-compliance
Lightning Source LLC
Chambersburg PA
CBHW051214290426
44109CB00021B/2448